AN INTRODUCTION TO
ELECTROCARDIOGRAPHY

AN INTRODUCTION TO
ELECTROCARDIOGRAPHY

by LEO SCHAMROTH

MD (Rand), DSc, FRCP (Edin),
FRCP (Glasg), FACC, FRS (SAf)

Professor of Medicine
University of the Witwatersrand
and Chief Physician
Baragwanath Hospital, Johannesburg
Republic of South Africa

SIXTH EDITION

BLACKWELL SCIENTIFIC PUBLICATIONS
OXFORD LONDON EDINBURGH
BOSTON MELBOURNE

First published 1957
Reprinted 1959, 1961
Second edition 1964
Third edition 1966
Reprinted 1968, 1969, 1970
Fourth edition 1973
Reprinted 1973, 1974
Fifth edition 1976
Reprinted 1978, 1980
Sixth edition 1982

Japanese translation 1966
Spanish translation 1974
Greek translation 1974
Italian translation 1980

Printed in Great Britain at
The Alden Press, Oxford
and bound by
Kemp Hall Bindery, Oxford

DISTRIBUTORS
USA
  Blackwell Mosby Book Distributors
  11830 Westline Industrial Drive
  St Louis, Missouri 63141

Canada
  Blackwell Mosby Book Distributors
  120 Melford Drive, Scarborough
  Ontario, M1B 2X4

Australia
  Blackwell Scientific Book
  Distributors
  214 Berkeley Street, Carlton
  Victoria 3053

British Library
Cataloguing in Publication Data

Schamroth, Leo
  An introduction to electrocardiography—6th ed.
  1. Electrocardiography
  I. Title
  616.1'207547   RC683.5.E5

ISBN 0–632–00973–X

TO THE MEMORY OF
BECKY

Contents

Foreword *by Professor G. A. Elliott*   xi

Preface to the Sixth Edition   xii

Preface to the First Edition   xiii

Acknowledgements   xiv

PART I. ABNORMALITIES OF THE P-QRS-T AND U DEFLECTIONS

Chapter

  1 Basic Principles   3

  2 Myocardial Death, Injury and Ischaemia   19

  3 Bundle Branch Block   72

  4 Ventricular Hypertrophy   80

  5 Drug and Electrolyte Effect   93

  6 The P Wave: Atrial Activation   101

  7 The Electrical Axis   106

  8 Hypothermia   139

  9 Electrical Alternans   140

10 The Q–T Interval   141

PART II. DISORDERS OF CARDIAC RHYTHM

SECTION 1. BASIC PRINCIPLES

11 Basic Principles   147

Contents

SECTION 2. DISORDERS OF IMPULSE FORMATION

12 Sinus Rhythms 154

13 Ectopic Atrial Rhythms 157

14 A-V Nodal Rhythms 171

15 Ventricular Rhythms 179

16 Parasystole 201

SECTION 3. DISORDERS OF IMPULSE CONDUCTION

17 Sino-atrial (S-A) Block 205

18 Atrioventricular (A-V) Block 207

19 Reciprocal Rhythm 221

20 The Supraventricular Tachycardias 228

21 The Wolff-Parkinson-White and Related
   Syndromes 233

SECTION 4. THE SECONDARY DISORDERS OF RHYTHM

22 Escape Rhythms 244

23 A-V Dissociation 249

24 Ventricular Fusion Complexes 255

25 Phasic Aberrant Ventricular Conduction 258

SECTION 5. CORRELATIVE ESSAY

26 Structural Nodal Disease: the So-Called Sick
   Sinus Syndrome 279

PART III. GENERAL CONSIDERATIONS AND CORRELATIVE OBSERVATIONS

27   General Observations and
     Correlative Observations   288

   The approach to electrocardiographic interpretation. Common
   associations. Common electrocardiographic manifestations of
   congenital heart disease. An approach to the diagnosis of
   arrhythmias. Form for routine reporting.

Appendix: Electrocardiographic Measurements   303

Index   314

Foreword

Dr Schamroth publishes this little book on modern electrocardiography at the insistent demand of students and graduates whom he
has instructed, and who consider that he should make available for
general circulation a method of teaching electrocardiography applicable to clinical practice which is simple, revealing and based upon
sound electro-physiological principles.

Simply written, and amply illustrated with many meaningful
diagrams, Dr Schamroth's book is a contribution to the rational
appreciation and interpretation of electrocardiographic abnormalities by students and practitioners whose training in the physiological
aspects of cardiac action has been no more profound than is provided
by the undergraduate curriculum.

Present-day literature on electrocardiography is forbidding in its
complexity for anyone who has not had specialized training. This
book is a welcome addition to electrocardiographic literature,
because by its simplicity and correctness it invites understanding.

G. A. Elliott
Professor of Medicine
University of the Witwatersrand

South Africa

Preface to the Sixth Edition

The basic design of this book remains essentially the same as that of the previous editions. It is directed primarily at the beginner, and its aim is simplicity. The emphasis remains on deductive rather than empirical electrocardiographic interpretation.

The whole text has been appreciably revised. New sections have been added on: ventricular fusion complexes, structural nodal disease—the so-called sick sinus syndrome, reciprocal rhythms, the supraventricular tachycardias, the Q–T interval and technical standardization. Many of the diagrams and illustrative electrocardiograms have been replaced, and new ones added.

L. Schamroth

Johannesburg, January 1982

Preface to the First Edition

This volume, it should be stated at the outset, makes no pretensions to be a complete or comprehensive treatise on electrocardiography, nor does it seek to supplant the major works on the subject. It is rather a stepping-stone to the fuller and more detailed study of a most important branch of medical science.

The student, introduced for the first time to the intricacies of electrocardiography, is frequently bewildered, sometimes overwhelmed, by complicated methods of presentation. It is the beginner who has been kept continuously in mind in the writing of this book, and the primary object throughout has been to give him a working knowledge of the subject. Consequently, a certain amount of licence has been taken with a view to clarifying the various processes. Theoretical considerations have been reduced to a minimum, emphasis being placed on the practical aspects. The text has been illustrated as profusely as possible with sketches, a clear drawing invariably being worth pages of script.

Clarity of presentation has thus been the author's aim; if he should succeed in dispersing a few clouds from his readers' minds, his efforts will not have been in vain.

L. Schamroth

Johannesburg, May 1956

Acknowledgements

It is my pleasure to express my thanks to:

Dr William P. Nelson for permission to reproduce his tracing as Fig. 169 in this text.

Dr A. Dubb for permission to reproduce his tracing as Fig. 93 in this text.

Mrs Catherine Marquard for permission to reproduce her tracing as Fig. 178.

Dr Hernandes Pieretti for permission to reproduce his tracing as Fig. 190.

The Photographic Department, Department of Medicine, University of the Witwatersrand, for the photographic reproductions.

PART I
ABNORMALITIES OF THE
P-QRS-T AND U
DEFLECTIONS

Basic Principles
Myocardial Death, Injury and Ischaemia
Bundle Branch Block
Ventricular Hypertrophy
Drug and Electrolyte Effect
The P Wave: Atrial Activation
The Electrical Axis
Hypothermia
Electrical Alternans
The Q–T Interval

Chapter 1
Basic Principles

THE ACTION OF THE GALVANOMETER

When an electrical impulse flows **towards** a unipolar electrode, or
the positive electrode of a bipolar lead, the galvanometer will record
a **positive** or upward deflection (Diagram A of Fig. 1).

When an electrical impulse flows **away** from a unipolar electrode,
or **away** from the positive electrode of a bipolar lead, i.e. towards the
negative pole of a bipolar electrode, the galvanometer will record a
negative or downward deflection (Diagram B of Fig. 1).

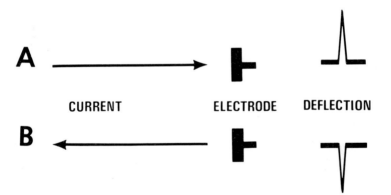

Fig. 1. Diagrams illustrating the effect of current direction on the positive electrodes
of a galvanometer.

THE 'TWO CHAMBER' CONCEPT

It is stating the obvious to say that the heart is a four-chambered
organ. It is not often appreciated, however, that, in an electrophysiological sense, the heart consists of only two chambers: one formed by
the atria, and the other formed by the ventricles (Fig. 2). The two
atria function as a single electrophysiological chamber—an electrophysiological unit: there is no electrical boundary between them, and
both are activated by a single activation process. This functional
electrophysiological unit may be referred to as the **bi-atrial**

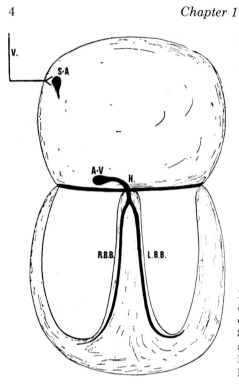

Fig. 2. Diagrammatic representation of the two electrophysiological chambers. V. = vagus nerve. S-A = sino-atrial node. A-V = atrioventricular node. H = bundle of His. R.B.B. = right bundle branch. L.B.B. = left bundle branch.

chamber. Similarly, the ventricles also function as an electrophysiological unit, which may be referred to as the **biventricular chamber.** The two electrophysiological chambers are separated from each other by an electrically inert conduction barrier formed by the fibrous A-V ring. Communication across this barrier under normal circumstances is only possible through the specialized conducting system formed by the A-V node, the bundle of His, the bundle branches and their ramifications.

THE DOMINANCE OF THE LEFT VENTRICLE

The free wall of the left ventricle, and the interventricular septum have relatively thick walls (large muscle masses) and together constitute a uniform ring of muscle or chamber—the anatomical left ventricle (Fig. 3). It is quite evident from a cross-section of the ventricles that the interventricular septum and the free wall of the left ventricle constitute an anatomical continuum (Fig. 3). The free wall of the right ventricle is, in effect, merely a thin anatomical appendage of the left ventricle.

The interventricular septum also contracts functionally with the free wall of the left ventricle, constituting the main haemodynamic pump of the heart. The right ventricle functions principally as a conduit.

From the electrocardiological viewpoint, the left ventricle is also the dominant chamber. For example, anterior wall myocardial infarction refers principally to infarction of the interventricular septum. The interventricular septum thus, in effect, constitutes the 'electrical' anterior wall of the biventricular chamber, whereas the thin free wall of the right ventricle constitutes the anatomical anterior wall of the biventricular chamber.

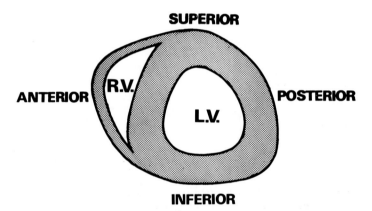

Fig. 3. Diagrammatic representation of a cross-section through the ventricles.

THE MODES OF ATRIAL AND VENTRICULAR ACTIVATION

The bi-atrial chamber is a relatively thin-walled structure and is not equipped with the highly specialized conducting system of the ventricles. Activation of the bi-atrial chamber therefore occurs **longitudinally** and by **contiguity,** spreading from its point of origin in the S-A node to engulf the whole chamber, each fibre in turn activating the adjacent fibre (Diagram A of Fig. 4).

Activation of the ventricles is effected through the specialized and highly efficient conducting system which transmits the supra-ventricular impulse very rapidly to all the endocardial regions of the chamber. The muscle is then activated from endocardial to epicardial surfaces through the terminal ramifications of the conducting system. Excitation therefore occurs **transversely** through the

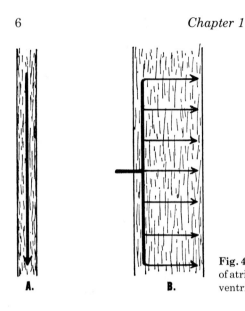

Fig. 4. Diagrams illustrating: (A) the mode of atrial activation. (B) the mode of ventricular activation.

A.   **B.**

ventricular myocardium, and this enables the whole chamber to be activated near-synchronously (Diagram B of Fig. 4).

These different forms of activation have both physiological and interpretative connotations. For example, atrial hypertrophy cannot be diagnosed electrocardiographically since the longitudinal form of atrial activation can only reflect *atrial enlargement.* The transverse form of ventricular activation, however, does permit electrocardiographic connotation with ventricular hypertrophy. The rapid near-synchronous transverse form of ventricular activation further means that the ventricles are rapidly brought to a similar electrophysiological state, i.e. uniform or a near-uniform. state of excitation or activation, and uniform or a near-uniform state of refractoriness. This constitutes one of the factors which militates against the development of ventricular fibrillation.

THE NOMENCLATURE OF THE ELECTROCARDIOGRAPHIC DEFLECTIONS

The electrocardiographic deflections are arbitrarily and sequentially named P, QRS, T and U. The P wave reflects atrial activation. The QRS complex reflects ventricular activation. The T wave reflects ventricular recovery. The genesis of the U wave is still controversial.

Note: An initial downward deflection after the P wave is termed a *q* wave. An initial upward deflection after the P wave is termed an *r* wave. The ensuing deflections are named by the succeeding alphabetical letters. Large, or relatively large, deflections are labelled with capital or upper-case alphabetic letters; small, or relatively small, deflections are labelled with non-capital, small or lower-case letters. Thus, a deep wide Q wave followed by a small r wave—as illustrated by Diagram C of Fig. 22—is labelled a Qr complex. A totally negative QRS deflection without ensuing positivity—as illustrated by Diagram D of Fig. 22—is labelled a QS complex. A small q wave followed by a tall or relatively tall R wave—as illustrated by Diagram A of Fig. 22—is labelled a qR complex. A small initial r wave followed by a deep or relatively deep S wave—as illustrated by lead V1 in Fig. 8—is labelled an rS complex. When the QRS complex reflects two positivities as occurs, for example, in right bundle branch block, the second positivity is termed an R', for example an rSR', an RsR', or an RR' complex.

ACTIVATION OF THE VENTRICLES

In an electrocardiological sense, the ventricles are composed of three muscle masses: the interventricular septum, the free wall of the right ventricle (the right ventricular muscle mass), the free wall of the left ventricle (the left ventricular muscle mass) (Fig. 5).

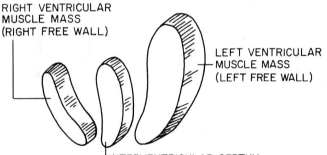

RIGHT VENTRICULAR MUSCLE MASS (RIGHT FREE WALL)

LEFT VENTRICULAR MUSCLE MASS (LEFT FREE WALL)

INTERVENTRICULAR SEPTUM

Fig. 5. The ventricular muscle masses.

In a simplified representation, activation—depolarization—of the ventricles begins in the left lower side of the interventricular septum and spreads through the septum from left to right (arrow 1 in Fig. 6).

Depolarization then proceeds outwards *simultaneously* and transversely through the free walls of both ventricles from endocardial to epicardial surfaces (arrows labelled 2 in Fig. 7).

The free wall of the left ventricle has a larger muscle mass—and hence a larger potential electrical force—than the free wall of the

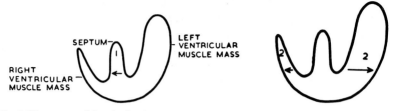

Fig. 6. First stage of depolarization.   **Fig. 7.** Second stage of depolarization.

right ventricle (Figs. 3 and 5). Consequently, as depolarization of both free walls occurs simultaneously, the larger left ventricular forces counteract the smaller right ventricular forces. The result is a single force directed from right to left (arrow 2 in Fig. 8). Thus, *for convenience*, depolarization of the ventricles may be represented in simplified form as a small initial force from left to right through the septum, followed by a larger force from right to left through the free wall of the left ventricle (Fig. 8). These forces have magnitude and direction and are thus vectors.

An electrode orientated to the left ventricle. (e.g. lead V6 in Fig. 8). will record a small initial downward deflection (a small q wave) caused by the spread of the stimulus *away* from the electrode through the septum, followed by a larger upward deflection (a tall R wave) caused by the spread of the stimulus *towards* the electrode through the left ventricular muscle mass (Fig. 8). The result is a qR complex (e.g. Standard lead I and leads V4 to V6 in Fig. 19; leads AVL, V5 and V6 in Fig. 77).

Conversely, an electrode orientated to the right ventricle (e.g. lead V1 in Fig. 8), will record a small initial upright deflection (a

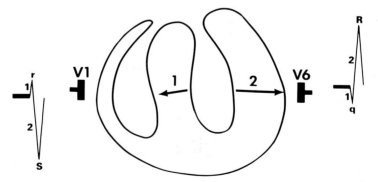

Fig. 8. Diagrammatic representation of the basic form of ventricular depolarization and its effect on leads V1 and V6.

small r wave) caused by the spread of the stimulus *towards* the electrode through the interventricular septum, followed by a larger downward deflection (a deep S wave) caused by the spread of the stimulus *away* from the electrode through the free wall of the left ventricular muscle mass (Fig. 8). The result is an rS complex (e.g. leads V1 and V2 in Fig. 19; leads V1 and V2 in Fig. 77).

NOMENCLATURE AND LOCATION OF THE ELECTRODE LEADS

Each electrocardiographic lead has a positive pole or electrode and a negative pole or electrode, which could theoretically be orientated in any relationship to the heart. By convention, however, there are 12 lead placements. These are:

> Standard lead I.
> Standard lead II.
> Standard lead III.
> Lead AVR.
> Lead AVL.
> Lead AVF.
> Leads V1 to V6.

Standard leads I, II and III are bipolar leads (see Appendix and Chapter 7).

Leads AVR, AVL, AVF and V1 to V6 are unipolar leads (see Appendix and Chapter 7).

BASIC ORIENTATION OF THE LEADS

The 12 conventional leads may be divided electrophysiologically into two groups, one being orientated in the frontal plane of the body, and the other in the horizontal plane (see Chapter 7 and Fig. 116).

Standard leads I, II and III, and leads AVR, AVL and AVF are orientated in the **frontal** or **coronal plane** of the body.

The precordial leads—leads V1 to V6—are orientated in the **horizontal** or **transverse plane** of the body.

The frontal plane leads

Standard leads I, II and III

The orientation of the Standard leads is described in Chapter 7.

Unipolar limb leads (see also Chapter 7).

All unipolar leads are termed V leads and consist of extremity or limb leads, and precordial or chest leads. Extremity leads are of low electrical potential and are therefore instrumentally augmented (see Appendix). These augmented extremity leads are thus prefixed by the letter 'A'.

Lead AVR is the augmented unipolar right arm lead (Fig. 9A). Electrically, the limbs may be viewed as extensions of the torso and it is immaterial whether the electrode is placed on the wrist, arm or shoulder. Thus lead AVR may be considered to be orientated to or 'face' the heart from the right shoulder (Fig. 9B). This lead is usually orientated to the cavity of the heart (see also page 122 and Fig. 117). Thus *all* the deflections—the P, QRS and T deflections—are normally negative in this lead (Fig. 19).

Lead AVL is the augmented unipolar left arm lead (Fig. 9A) and may be considered to be orientated to or to 'face' the heart from the left shoulder (Fig. 9B). This lead is usually orientated to the anterolateral or superior surface of the left ventricle.

Lead AVF is the augmented unipolar left leg lead (Fig. 9A) and may be considered to be orientated to the inferior surface of the heart (Fig. 9B).

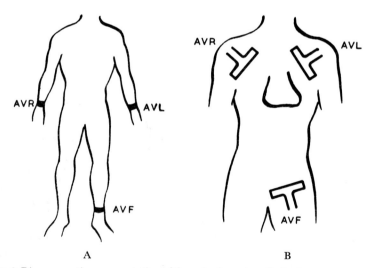

Fig. 9. Diagrammatic representation of the unipolar extremity leads.

The horizontal plane leads

PRECORDIAL OR CHEST LEADS

The precordial leads are designated by the letter 'V' as the only alphabetical letter (Figs. 10 and 11).

Lead V1 is located over the fourth intercostal space to the right of the sternal border.

Lead V2 is located over the fourth intercostal space to the left of the sternal border.

Lead V3 is located midway between leads V2 and V4.

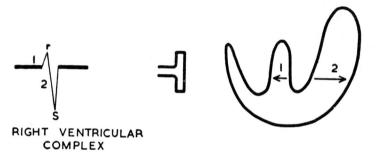

RIGHT VENTRICULAR
COMPLEX

Fig. 10. Diagrammatic representation of the precordial leads.

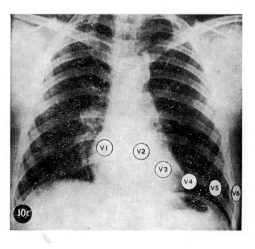

Fig. 11. The precordial leads and their relationship to the heart and thorax.

Lead V4 is located on the midclavicular line over the fifth interspace.

Lead V5 is located on the anterior axillary line at the same level as lead V4.

Lead V6 is located over the midaxillary line at the same level as leads V4 and V5.

Orientation of the electrocardiographic leads to the left ventricular 'cone'

Since the left ventricle is the dominant electrophysiological chamber of the heart, orientation of the electrodes to this chamber is of particular importance. The left ventricle is in the form of a cone whose apex is directed downward and to the left (Fig. 12). It has five surfaces or regions each with a specific lead orientation (Table 1).

THE ELECTROCARDIOGRAPHIC REFLECTION OF THE SO-CALLED ANATOMICAL HEART POSITION

'ROTATION' OF THE HEART

It was previously thought that the anatomical orientation of the heart could vary under both normal and pathological conditions, and that this could be reflected electrocardiographically. It is very doubtful, however, whether true anatomical movement does indeed

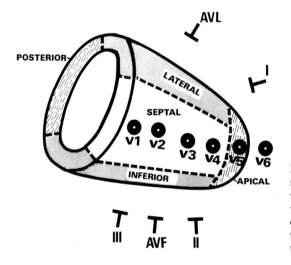

Fig. 12. Diagrammatic representation of the various surfaces of the left ventricular anatomical cone, and their relationship to the frontal and horizontal plane leads.

Table 1. Left ventricle surfaces and lead orientations.

Surface or region	Lead orientation
1. Anteroseptal	Leads V1 to V4.
2. Anterolateral or superior	Standard lead I and lead AVL.
3. Inferior	Standard leads II and III, and lead AVF.
4. Posterior	No direct lead orientation. Diagnosis of abnormality in this region is made from inverse or 'mirror-image' changes in leads V1 to V3.
5. Apical	Leads V5 and V6.

occur. It is far more likely that so-called clockwise and counter-clockwise rotation, and horizontal and vertical heart positions reflect changes in mean frontal and horizontal plane electrical axes—a change in the orientation of the mean electrical force rather than a change in anatomical position. Nevertheless, the terms are still in use, and the concept is presented here for didactic purposes with the aforementioned reservation in mind.

The heart can theoretically 'rotate' around two hypothetical axes: the *anteroposterior axis* and the *oblique or longitudinal axis*. 'Rotation' around the anteroposterior axis reflects rotation in the frontal plane. 'Rotation' around the oblique or longitudinal axis reflects rotation in the horizontal plane.

'Rotation' in the frontal plane

The anteroposterior axis theoretically runs through the septum of the heart from anterior to posterior surfaces (Fig. 13). Rotation around this axis will result in a so-called horizontal or vertical heart position, and is diagnosed from the presence of a dominantly positive QRS deflection or qR complex in lead AVL or lead AVF.

'HORIZONTAL' POSITION

In the 'horizontal' position the main muscle mass of the left ventricle is orientated upwards and to the left, i.e. towards lead AVL and the positive pole of Standard lead I (Fig. 14). These leads will therefore record a qR or 'left ventricular' complex (e.g. lead AVL in Fig. 77).

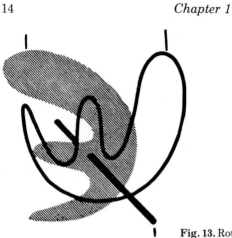

Fig. 13. Rotation round the anteroposterior axis.

'VERTICAL' POSITION

In the 'vertical' position the main muscle mass of the left ventricle is orientated downwards and to the left, i.e. towards lead AVF and the positive pole of Standard lead II (Fig. 15). These leads will therefore record a qR or 'left ventricular' complex (e.g. lead AVF in Fig. 79).

SUMMARY

A qR complex in lead AVL and Standard lead I indicates a **'horizontal'** heart position.

A qR complex in lead AVF and Standard lead II indicates a **'vertical'** heart position.

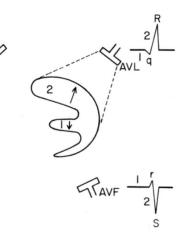

Fig. 14. The so-called horizontal heart position—a qR complex in lead AVL.

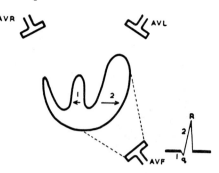

Fig. 15. Vertical position of the heart.

COMMENT

It must be stressed once again that it is doubtful whether any significant movement or rotation does, in fact, occur in this plane. 'Horizontality' of the heart, however, most likely reflects left axis deviation; and this is not the expression of heart movement, but rather an intraventricular conduction defect (see Chapter 7). A 'vertical' heart position most likely reflects an inferiorly or rightwardly directed QRS axis.

'Rotation' in the horizontal plane

The oblique or longitudinal axis of the heart runs obliquely from the apex to the base of the heart (Fig. 16). Rotation round this axis is conventionally viewed from below the heart looking towards the apex and will result in clockwise or counter-clockwise movement. This is diagnosed from the precordial leads.

CLOCKWISE ROTATION

Clockwise rotation round the oblique axis will cause the right ventricle to assume a more anterior position. The right ventricle and interventricular septum will lie parallel to and face the anterior chest wall and the V leads (Fig 17). Thus, all the conventional precordial leads—leads VI to V6—are orientated to the right ventricle and record rS or 'right ventricular' complexes (Fig. 83).

COUNTER-CLOCKWISE ROTATION

Counter-clockwise rotation round the oblique axis of the heart causes the left ventricle to rotate a few degrees anteriorly so that

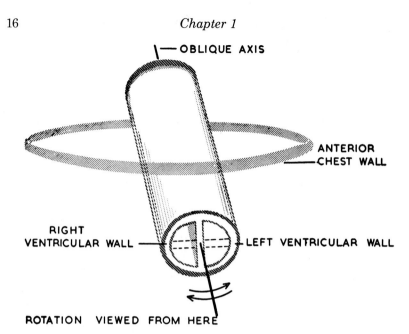

Fig. 16. Diagrammatic representation of the heart with the apex removed, to show rotation round the oblique axis.

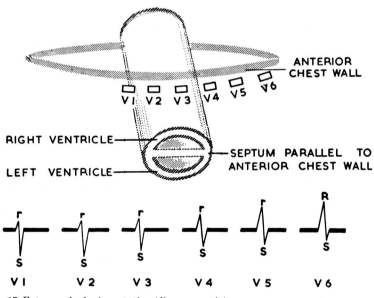

Fig. 17. Extreme clockwise rotation (diagrammatic).

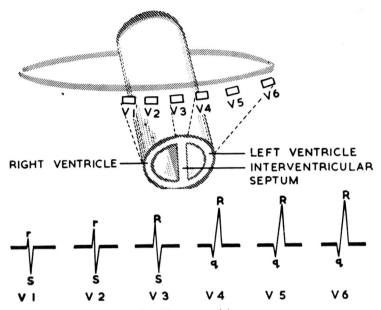

Fig. 18. Counter-clockwise rotation (diagrammatic).

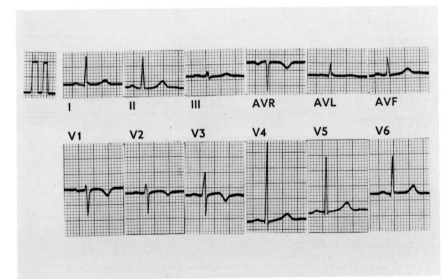

Fig. 19. Normal electrocardiogram. *Note*: 1. The normal standardization (see Appendix, page 299). 2. Leads V1 and V2 are orientated to the right ventricle and reflect rS complexes. 3. Leads V4 to V6 are orientated to the left ventricle and reflect qR complexes. 4. Lead V3 reflects the transition zone. 5. Lead V6 resembles Standard lead I. 6. All the deflections in lead AVR are negative.

both right and left ventricles face the anterior chest wall and the precordial leads (Fig. 18). As a result, leads V1 to V3 face the right ventricle and record rS complexes; leads V4 to V6 face the left ventricle and record qR complexes (Fig. 76). The area of change from rS to qR pattern is known as the **transition zone** (e.g. lead V3 in Fig. 19). See also comment on the transition zone on page 298.

SUMMARY

Clockwise rotation: rS complexes in lead V1 to V6.
Counter-clockwise rotation: rS complexes in leads V1, V2, (V3), qR complexes in leads (V3), V4, V5, V6.

STANDARDIZATION

The technical standardization of the electrocardiograph and the electrocardiographic effects of incorrect standardization are considered in the Appendix page 299.

Chapter 2
Myocardial Death, Injury
and Ischaemia

MYOCARDIAL INFARCTION

Myocardial infarction is reflected electrocardiographically by the electrocardiographic parameters of *Necrosis, injury* and *ischaemia*. The infarction process progresses through three phases:
1. **An early 'hyperacute' phase.**
2. **A fully evolved phase.**
3. **A phase of resolution.**

The principles governing the electrocardiographic manifestations of necrosis, injury and ischaemia are best understood and illustrated with reference to the fully evolved phase, and this will therefore be considered first.

THE FULLY EVOLVED PHASE OF ACUTE MYOCARDIAL INFARCTION

THE ELECTROCARDIOGRAPHIC MANIFESTATION OF MYOCARDIAL NECROSIS

Myocardial necrosis is reflected by a **deep and wide Q wave** or a QS complex by electrodes orientated towards the necrotic area.

Mechanism

Dead tissue is electrically inert and cannot be activated or depolarized. If the dead tissue involves practically the full thickness of the muscle wall it constitutes a transmural infarct (Diagram A of Fig. 20) and there is, in an electrical sense, a 'hole' or 'window' in the muscle wall (Diagram B of Fig. 20).

An electrode orientated to or placed over this 'hole' reflects activity of distant healthy muscle as 'seen' through the 'window' (Fig. 21).

Thus, an electrode placed over an area of dead muscle in the left ventricular wall reflects: first, septal depolarization—a negative

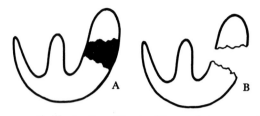

Fig. 20. (A) Diagrammatic illustration of the dead tissue of a transmural infarct. (B) The 'electrical hole' or 'window' created by the dead tissue.

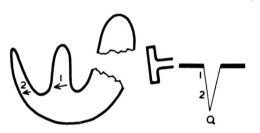

Fig. 21. Diagram illustrating the electrocardiographic effect on an electrode orientated to the electrical 'hole' resulting from infarction of the free wall of the left ventricle.

deflection (arrow 1 in Fig. 21) and, secondly, distant right ventricular depolarization—a further negative deflection (arrow 2 in Fig. 21). This results in an initial broad deep Q wave—the pathological Q wave of myocardial infarction, or a QS complex (Fig. 21, Diagrams C of Figs. 22 and 25; and, for example, leads V2, V3 and V4 of Fig. 30).

Note: An entirely negative deflection without an ensuing R wave is sometimes termed a QS deflection. (Diagram D of Fig. 22; Diagram C of Fig. 25.)

This phenomenon may also be interpreted vectorially, in the sense that **electrical forces are directed away from a necrotic or infarcted area** (see also Chapter 7, page 128).

Furthermore, if the necrosis is not transmural and there is surviving viable myocardial tissue, the amplitude of the R wave will be diminished in leads orientated to the infarcted area. This principle is illustrated in Fig. 22. Diagram A of Fig. 22 reflects normal muscle tissue and normal endocardial to epicardial activation. The resulting R wave will be of normal amplitude. Diagram B of Fig. 22 reflects minimal subendocardial necrosis, and the resulting R wave is likewise unchanged. Diagram C illustrates the effect of significant subendocardial necrosis. This results in (*a*) a significant loss of initial forces, as evidenced by a pathological Q wave, and (*b*) late activation

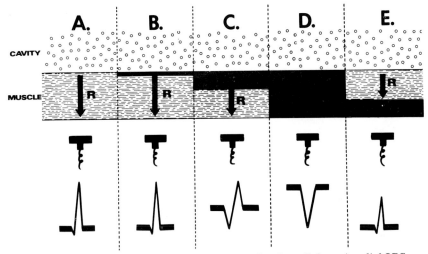

Fig. 22. Diagrammatic illustration of: (A) the normal endocardial to epicardial QRS activation; (B) the hypothetical unchanged QRS activation associated with minimal subendocardial necrosis; (C) the diminished QRS activation (following a pathological Q wave) associated with significant subendocardial necrosis; (D) the absent QRS activation associated with transmural necrosis and (E) the diminished QRS activation associated with subepicardial necrosis.

of the overlying viable tissue resulting in the inscription of a terminal r or R wave. A lead orientated to this region will thus reflect a Qr or QR complex. This is exemplified by lead V5 in Fig. 30 and Standard leads II and III, and lead AVF in Fig. 42. Diagram D reflects transmural necrosis, resulting in a total loss of forces orientated to the facing electrode which, therefore, records a totally negative or QS complex. Diagram E reflects epicardial necrosis. This will result in diminished amplitude of the R wave but no initial pathological Q wave in a lead orientated to this region. This is exemplified by leads V5 and V6 in Fig. 39.

THE ELECTROCARDIOGRAPHIC MANIFESTATION OF MYOCARDIAL INJURY

Myocardial injury is reflected electrocardiographically by **deviation of the S-T segment.** The S-T segment is, so to speak, *deviated towards the surface of the injured tissue.* Thus, if the injury is dominantly epicardial (as illustrated in Diagram A of Fig. 23), the S-T segment is deviated towards the injured epicardial surface, and a lead orientated towards this surface (e.g. lead V6 in Diagram A of Fig. 23)

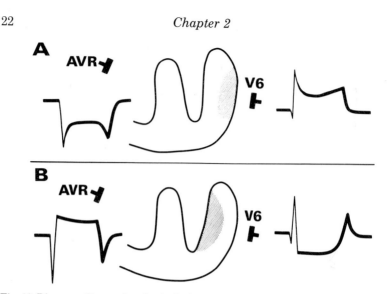

Fig. 23. Diagrams illustrating the deviation of the S-T segment in: (A) dominant subepicardial injury, and (B) dominant subendocardial injury.

will reflect a raised S-T segment. Conversely, a lead orientated towards the uninjured surface (e.g. lead AVR in Diagram A of Fig. 23) will reflect a depressed S-T segment. With a dominantly subendocardial injury, a lead orientated to the injured subendocardial surface (e.g. lead AVR in Diagram B of Fig. 23) will reflect an elevated S-T segment, whereas a lead orientated to the uninjured surface (lead V6 in Diagram B of Fig. 23) will reflect a depressed S-T segment; see also Fig. 48.

Since the myocardial injury in most infarctions is dominantly epicardial with some subendocardial 'sparing' (Fig. 24), the manifestation presents electrocardiographically with elevated S-T segments in leads orientated to the epicardial surface. The S-T segments in the fully evolved phase of the infarction are, in addition, *coved or convex-upward*.

The mechanism of these S-T segment shifts is still controversial. Several theories have been propounded, one of which is considered in the Appendix (page 305).

THE ELECTROCARDIOGRAPHIC EFFECTS OF MYOCARDIAL ISCHAEMIA

Myocardial ischaemia is reflected by an inverted T wave in leads orientated to the ischaemic surface. Inverted T waves are, however, non-specific and may be associated with many other conditions both normal and abnormal. However, the T waves associated with myocardial ischaemia have certain characteristics which tend to reflect their 'ischaemic' origin. They are usually **'arrowhead'** in appearance being *peaked, symmetrical* and increased in magnitude (e.g. leads V2 to V6 in Fig. 30).

THE COMBINED PATTERNS OF THE FULLY EVOLVED PHASE OF MYOCARDIAL INFARCTION

A severely infarcted area consists of necrotic tissue surrounded by a zone of injured tissue which, in turn, is surrounded by a zone of ischaemic tissue (Fig. 24).

A conventional electrode cannot be pinpointed or placed directly over the heart muscle itself; it is situated some distance away and therefore subtends a relatively large area to include the zones of necrotic, injured and ischaemic tissues (Fig. 24). Such an electrode will record all three patterns, viz. the pathological Q wave, the raised coved S-T segment and the inverted, pointed symmetrical arrowhead T wave (Diagram C of Fig. 25 and leads V2 to V4 in Fig. 30). This will be referred to as the *typical infarction pattern.*

An electrode orientated towards injured and ischaemic tissue but

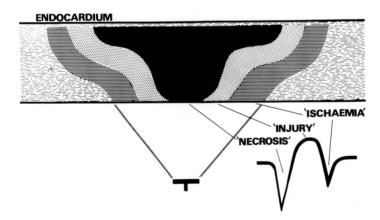

Fig. 24. An idealized representation of the combined patterns of the fully evolved phase of acute myocardial infarction. The infarct is pyramid-shaped with a broad base towards the endocardium. The diagram also illustrates the hypothetical 'rind' of subendocardial 'sparing' (see Appendix, page 306). Note that 'necrosis', 'injury' and 'ischaemia' are in quotation marks since they do not precisely represent their pathologic counterparts but rather reflect a progressive loss of potassium from the cell.

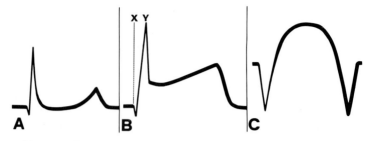

Fig. 25. Diagrams illustrating: (A) normal QRST complex, (B) the hyperacute phase of myocardial infarction, and (C) the fully evolved phase of myocardial infarction. Interval X–Y represents the increased ventricular activation time.

not necrotic tissue will record the raised, coved S-T segment and the inverted pointed symmetrical T wave only. The pathological Q wave may be absent or relatively insignificant. The amplitude of the R wave, however, is frequently diminished, thereby also reflecting a loss of viable tissue (e.g. lead V6 of Fig. 30).

Note: Reciprocal depression of the S-T segment will occur in leads orientated towards the uninjured surface. These are termed reciprocal changes. However, the diagnosis of infarction must not be based on depressed S-T segments only, as these may occur in conditions such as angina pectoris (see page 46). *The diagnosis must be based on pathological Q waves and/or the typically raised and coved S-T segments.* These are termed indicative changes.

THE HYPERACUTE PHASE OF MYOCARDIAL INFARCTION

The hyperacute phase of myocardial infarction occurs within a few hours of the onset of myocardial infarction. It was so named to distinguish it from the well-recognized fully evolved phase of myocardial infarction, as described earlier in this chapter. The condition has received insufficient emphasis in the electrocardiographic literature. Furthermore, since the transition to the fully evolved phase occurs relatively early—usually within 24 hours—the manifestation is not infrequently missed. Thus, the first electrocardiogram of the patient is often recorded during the fully evolved phase. Yet, the hyperacute phase is probably the most important and critical developmental stage of the infarction process, for it is then that the complication of primary ventricular fibrillation is most likely to occur. In other words, the manifestation of the hyperacute phase is an indication for intense vigilance and the necessity for coronary care monitoring.

ELECTROCARDIOGRAPHIC MANIFESTATIONS

The hyperacute phase of myocardial infarction is characterized by four principal electrocardiographic manifestations in leads orientated to the infarcted surface (Diagram B of Fig. 25, and Figs. 26, 27 and 28):

1. Slope-elevation of the S-T segment.
2. Tall and widened T waves.
3. Increased ventricular activation time.
4. Increased amplitude of the R wave.

1. *Slope-elevation of the S-T segment*

The S-T segment in the hyperacute phase is elevated—often markedly so—and has a straight upward slope to the apex of the T wave. The slope may, at times, also be slightly concave-upward. The S-T segment thus blends smoothly and imperceptibly with the proximal limb of the tall and widened T wave (see below). (Figs. 25, 26, 27 and 28.) The proximal limb of the T wave, in effect, constitutes the elevated S-T segment.

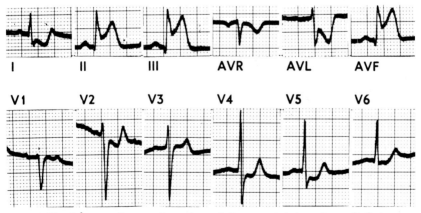

Fig. 26. The electrocardiogram shows the early hyperacute injury phase of inferior wall myocardial infarction. This is reflected by the marked slope-elevation of the S-T segments, and the increased amplitude of the T waves in Standard leads II and III, and lead AVF. Reciprocal S-T segment depression occurs in Standard leads I, lead AVL and leads V4 to V6.

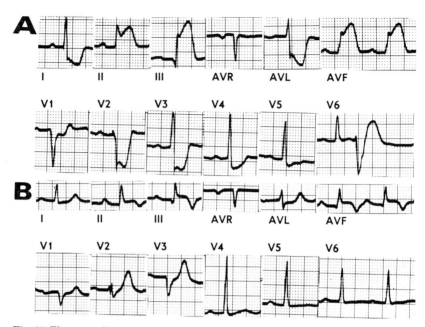

Fig. 27. Electrocardiogram A was recorded on admission to the coronary care unit, and shows the hyperacute early injury phase of acute inferior wall myocardial infarction. This is reflected by the following:

(*a*) There is marked slope-elevation of the S-T segments in Standard leads II and III, and lead AVF.

(*b*) There is an increase in the amplitude of the R wave in Standard leads II and III, and lead AVF (compare with Electrocardiogram B).

(*c*) There is an increase in ventricular activation time, as reflected by a delay in the inscription of the intrinsicoid deflection to 0.06 sec; best seen in Standard lead III and lead AVF.

(*d*) There is a reciprocal depression of the S-T segment in leads V1 to V5, Standard lead I and lead AVL.

(*e*) The single ventricular extrasystole in lead V6 reflects a primary S-T segment change. This is reflected by the upward coving of the S-T segment instead of the straight or minimally concave-upward secondary S-T segment change of an uncomplicated ventricular extrasystole.

(*f*) The low to inverted T waves in leads V5 and V6 reflect a lateral extension of the myocardial ischaemia.

(*g*) There is first-degree A-V block, the P–R interval measures 0.24 sec.

Electrocardiogram B was recorded 2 days later when the patient no longer had any chest pain and shows the fully evolved phase of acute inferior wall myocardial infarction. This is reflected by the following:

(*a*) The S-T segments are coved and elevated, and the T waves are inverted, sharply pointed and arrowhead in appearance in Standard leads II and III, and lead AVF.

(*b*) Standard lead III has a pathological Q wave.

(*c*) The T waves are low to inverted in leads V5 and V6, representing some lateral, apical, extension of the myocardial ischaemia.

(*d*) Standard lead I, lead AVL and leads V1 to V3 reflect reciprocal, symmetrical and widened T waves.

(*e*) There is first degree A-V block, the P–R interval measures 0.24 sec.

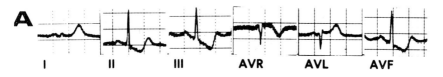

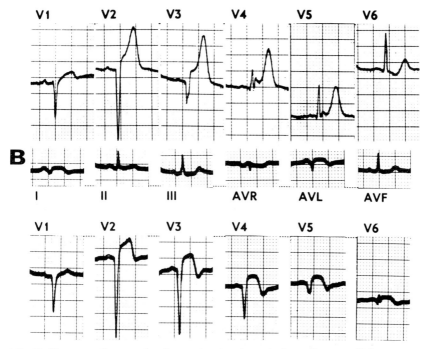

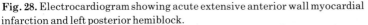

Fig. 28. Electrocardiogram showing acute extensive anterior wall myocardial infarction and left posterior hemiblock.

Electrocardiogram A shows the very early hyperacute phase of acute anterior wall myocardial infarction. This is reflected by the very tall T waves in leads V2 to V6, Standard lead I and lead AVL. There is also a degree of slope-elevation of the S-T segments in leads V2 to V4 and lead AVL.

Standard leads II and III, and lead AVF reflect reciprocal depression of the S-T segments. This is the mirror-image pattern of the S-T segment slope-elevation and the inverted T waves.

The QS complexes of myocardial necrosis are present in leads V2 and V3, reflecting a loss of the initial positivity. Note that the initial small r wave is still present in lead V1, but has disappeared in leads V2 and V3.

Note: Very tall and wide T waves are, at times, the earliest and most striking manifestations of acute myocardial infarction.

Electrocardiogram B was recorded on the following day and shows the fully evolved phase of the acute extensive anterior wall myocardial infarction. The parameters of myocardial necrosis are reflected by the QS complexes in leads V1 to V5, Standard lead I and lead AVL, and the pathological Q wave of the Qr complex in lead V6. The parameters of myocardial injury and ischaemia are reflected by the coved and elevated S-T segments and inverted, symmetrical T waves in leads V2 to V6, Standard lead I and lead AVL.

The left posterior hemiblock is reflected by the mean frontal plane QRS axis of +90° to +100°.

Leads orientated to the uninjured surface usually reflect marked reciprocal S-T segment depression.

2. *Tall and widened T wave*

The T wave becomes appreciably taller and may approach, or at times even exceed, the height of the R wave (Figs. 25, 26, 27 and 28). The T wave also becomes widened, and its proximal limb blends with the elevated S-T segment (see above), so that the two components cannot be separated. These very tall T waves may, at times, be the dominant feature of the hyperacute phase of myocardial infarction (Fig. 28). The differential diagnosis of tall precordial T waves is considered on page 297.

The classic pathological Q wave of myocardial infarction does not occur until this large amplitude upright T wave has regressed.

3. *Increased ventricular activation time*

There is an increase in the ventricular activation time, i.e. a delay in the onset of the intrinsicoid deflection: the time from the beginning of the QRS complex to the apex of the R wave (interval X–Y in Diagram B of Fig. 25; see also Fig. 241).

This manifestation is due to a degree of intraventricular— injury—block: the activation process takes longer to travel through the injured though still viable infarcted region.

4. *Increased amplitude of the R wave*

This is particularly seen with the hyperacute phase of inferior wall myocardial infarction.

Note: The hyperacute phase of myocardial infarction is analogous to the electrocardiographic manifestation of the variant form of angina pectoris where it occurs as a transient phenomenon (see page 50).

LOCALIZATION OF INFARCTED AREAS

Infarcts occur predominantly in the anterior, inferior (or diaphragmatic) and posterior, walls of the left ventricle (Figs. 29, 31, 33, 35, 37 and 38; see also Fig. 12).

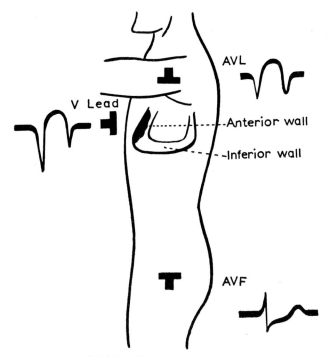

Fig. 29. Anterior myocardial infarction.

ANTERIOR WALL INFARCTION

The anterior surface of the left ventricle is orientated towards the precordial leads (Figs. 29 and 37); the anterolateral surface of the left ventricle is orientated towards lead AVL and the positive pole of Standard lead I (Fig 118; see also Fig. 12). Thus, anterior infarcts will be reflected by the presence of the typical infarction pattern—pathological Q wave, raised S-T segment and inverted T wave—in Standard Lead I, lead AVL and the precordial leads (Figs. 30 and 31).

Anterior infarcts may be further arbitrarily divided into **extensive anterior infarction** (Figs. 30 and 31); **anteroseptal infarction** (Figs. 31 and 32); and **anterolateral infarction** (Figs. 31, 33 and 34).

An **extensive anterior infarction** is reflected by the typical infarction pattern in Standard lead I, lead AVL and *all* the precordial leads (Figs. 28, 30 and 31).

An **anteroseptal infarction** is an infarction across the interventricular septum and is reflected by the typical infarction pattern in leads V1 to V4 (Figs. 31 and 32).

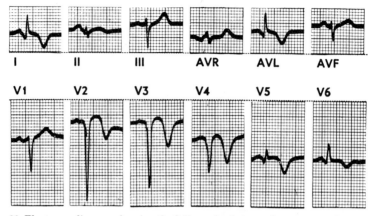

Fig. 30. Electrocardiogram showing the fully evolved phase of acute extensive anterior myocardial infarction. Note the typical infarction pattern of the fully evolved phase of acute myocardial infarction in leads V2 to V6, AVL and Standard lead I.

An **anterolateral infarction** is reflected by the typical infarction pattern in leads I, AVL, and in leads V4 to V6 (Figs. 31, 33 and 34).

INFERIOR—DIAPHRAGMATIC—INFARCTION

Lead AVF and the positive poles of Standard Leads II and III are orientated to the inferior or diaphragmatic surface of the heart (Figs. 35 and 37). Thus, inferior wall infarcts will be reflected by the presence of the typical infarction pattern—pathological Q wave, raised S-T segment and inverted T wave—in leads II, III and AVF (Figs. 27, 34, 36, 39 and 124).

TRUE POSTERIOR WALL INFARCTION

Infarction of the true posterior wall of the left ventricle is uncommon

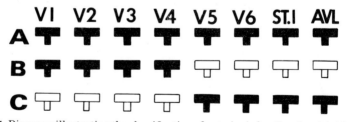

Fig. 31. Diagrams illustrating the classification of anterior infarction. Leads with the blackened electrodes reflect the infarction pattern. (A) Extensive anterior infarction. (B) Anteroseptal infarction. (C) Anterolateral infarction.

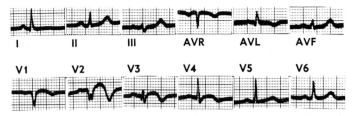

Fig. 32. Electrocardiogram showing the fully evolved phase of anteroseptal infarction. This is reflected by the pathological Q waves in leads V1 to V3, the coved elevated S-T segments and the inverted T waves in leads V1 to V4.

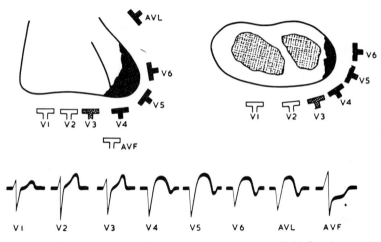

Fig. 33. The fully evolved phase of acute anterolateral myocardial infarction.

and manifests with distinctive electrocardiographic features which are strikingly different from the usual infarction pattern. The classic electrocardiographic features of the fully evolved phase of acute myocardial infarction, viz. deep and wide Q wave, elevated and coved S-T segment and inverted arrowhead T wave, which manifest in the conventional leads orientated to the infarcted surface, do not occur. This is because none of these leads is orientated towards the true posterior surface of the heart. The diagnosis of true posterior infarction is thus made from 'inverse' changes in leads which are orientated towards the uninjured—anterior—surface of the heart, viz. leads V1, V2 and V3 (see also Fig. 12).

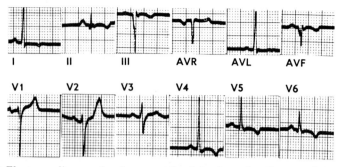

Fig. 34. Electrocardiogram showing regressing inferolateral wall myocardial infarction. The electrocardiogram was recorded 3 weeks after the onset of acute myocardial infarction. The necrosis of the inferior wall is reflected by the pathological Q waves in Standard lead III and lead AVF as well as the prominent q wave in Standard lead II. The myocardial injury and ischaemia are reflected by the slightly elevated and coved S-T segments, and the inverted T waves in Standard leads II and III, and lead AVF. The anterolateral extension is reflected by the coved S-T segments and inverted T waves in leads V4 to V6 and Standard lead I, as well as the inverted T wave in lead AVL.

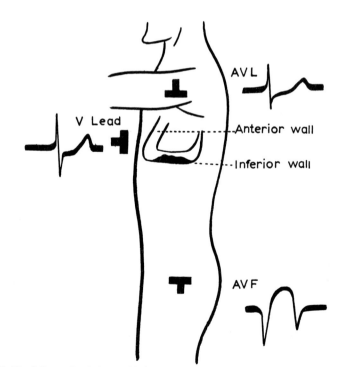

Fig. 35. The fully evolved phase of inferior wall myocardial infarction.

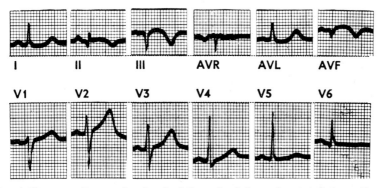

Fig. 36. Electrocardiogram showing the fully evolved phase of acute inferior wall myocardial infarction. Note the typical infarction pattern in Standard leads II and III, and lead AVF. Leads AVL and Standard I show reciprocal S-T segment depression. The T waves are low in leads V5 and V6 suggesting some anterolateral extension.

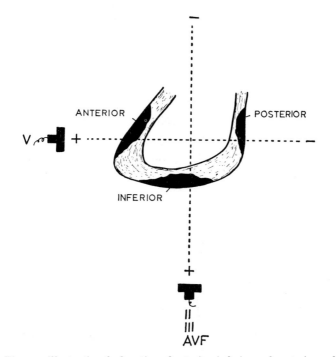

Fig. 37. Diagram illustrating the location of anterior, inferior and posterior wall myocardial infarctions.

Electrocardiographic manifestations of true posterior wall infarction

True posterior infarction manifests electrocardiographically with:
1. *Tall and slightly widened R waves in leads V1, V2 and V3.*[4, 32]
2. *Tall, wide and symmetrical T waves in leads V1, V2 and V3.*
The genesis of these changes is considered below.

1. *Tall and slightly widened R waves in leads V1, V2 and V3*[4, 32]

Depolarization of the normal heart begins in the lower left side of the interventricular septum and spreads from left to right—and anteriorly—through the septum (Vector 1 in Diagram A of Fig. 38). This is followed by simultaneous activation from endocardial to epicardial surfaces of the free walls of the right (anterior) and left (posterior) ventricles (Vectors 2 in Diagram A of Fig. 38). Since, however, the left or posterior wall has a larger muscle mass, and hence a larger potential electrical force, its activation force will counteract the

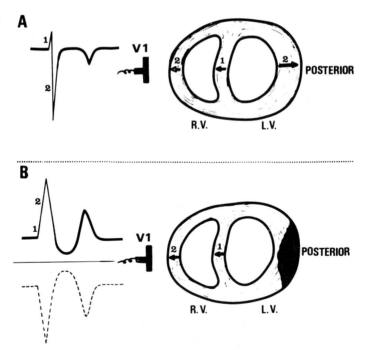

Fig. 38. Diagrams illustrating (A) normal ventricular depolarization and (B) ventricular depolarization during true posterior wall infarction (see text).

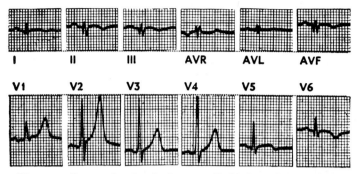

| I | II | III | AVR | AVL | AVF |

| V1 | V2 | V3 | V4 | V5 | V6 |

Fig. 39. Electrocardiogram showing the features of inferolateral myocardial infarction with true posterior extension. The fully evolved phase of myocardial infarction is seen in Standard leads II and III, and lead AVF, indicating the presence of an inferior wall infarction. The infarction pattern is also seen in lead V6 indicating lateral wall extension. The tall R wave and tall symmetrical T wave in leads V1, V2 and V3 indicates true posterior extension.

small force of the right (anterior) ventricle which is opposite in direction. This is reflected in leads V1 and V2 by a small initial r wave—caused by the 'septal' force which is directed toward the electrode, followed by a deep S wave resulting from the left or posterior wall force moving away from the electrode.

When the posterior wall is infarcted, the left or posterior wall force is lost (Diagram B of Fig. 38). Thus, activation of the interventricular septum (Vector 1 in Diagram B of Fig. 38) is followed by activation of the free or anterior wall of the right ventricle. Both forces are now orientated towards leads V1 and V2 resulting in tall and widened R waves in these leads (Fig. 39). This may also be expressed as an increase in the R/S ratio to greater than 1 (normal being less than 1). This manifestation is, in effect, a mirror-image of the pathologic Q wave which would be recorded by an electrode orientated towards the posterior surface of the heart (dotted lines in Diagram B of Fig. 38).

There are, however, other conditions which give rise to tall R waves in leads V1 and V2 which must be excluded before the diagnosis of true posterior infarction can be established with certainty. These are:

(a) *Right ventricular dominance* (see page 83).
(b) *The Wolff-Parkinson-White syndrome* (see page 235).
(c) *Certain forms of right bundle branch block.*
(d) *Mirror image dextrocardia.*
(e) *Normal variant.*

(*a*) Right ventricular dominance is reflected by right axis deviation, associated right atrial enlargement and the T waves are usually
inverted in the right precordial leads (see Chapter 4). There will
usually be corroborative clinical evidence of right ventricular
dominance.

(*b*) The Wolff-Parkinson-White syndrome will reflect the classic
features of short P–R interval, delta wave and secondary S-T segment
and T wave changes (see Chapter 21).

(*c*) Right bundle branch block will reflect the RsR′ pattern in
leads orientated to the right ventricle, and a qRS pattern in leads
orientated to the left ventricle (see Chapter 3).

(*d*) Mirror-image dextrocardia. This will be reflected by: (i) Tall R
waves in the right precordial leads with diminishing amplitude
towards the left, and (ii) rightward deviation of the P, QRS and T
wave axes, i.e. the P wave, QRS complex and T wave will be inverted
in Standard lead I and Lead AVL.

(*e*) Normal variant. A relatively tall R wave may at times appear
as a normal variant in the right precordial leads. This is always
associated with a terminal S wave. In other words, the normal variant
always manifests as an RS complex.

Note that in none of the aforementioned five conditions will there
be an associated tall upright and widened T wave.

2. *Tall, upright, and symmetrical T waves in leads V1, V2 and V3*

The T wave vector is always directed away from the area of
infarction. Thus, in true posterior infarction, the T wave vector is
directed anteriorly, resulting in tall, symmetrical T waves in leads V1
and V2 (Fig. 39).

This tall symmetrical widened and upright T wave is a characteristic of true posterior wall infarction, and the diagnosis should not be
entertained without it. The differential diagnosis of tall precordial T
waves is considered on page 290.

The theoretical question of S-T segment depression in leads V1, V2 and V3

In acute myocardial infarction, the S-T segment vector shifts towards
the injured surface, i.e. to leads orientated to the injured surface
which reflect elevated and coved S-T segments. In the case of true
posterior infarction, the S-T segment vector will thus, theoretically,
shift away from leads orientated towards the anterior surface of the

heart and thereby, theoretically, resulting in depressed and concave-upward S-T segments in leads V1, V2 and V3. However, this is rarely, if ever, seen.

THE 'INVERSE' CHANGES

The combination of tall R waves and tall, widened symmetrical T waves in the right precordial leads occurring in true posterior myocardial infarction is, in effect, the mirror-image of the typical infarction pattern which would be recorded by a lead orientated towards the true posterior wall (Fig. 39). The tall R wave is the mirror-image of the pathologic Q wave (Fig. 40), the depressed S-T segment is the mirror-image of the elevated S-T segment, and the tall, symmetrical T wave is the mirror-image of the deeply inverted T wave (dotted line in Diagram B of Fig. 38).

Note. True posterior infarction rarely, if ever, occurs as an isolated manifestation, but is usually associated with inferior and/or apico-lateral infarction.

THE PHASE OF RESOLUTION

Resolution of the electrocardiographic pattern of acute myocardial infarction progresses from the fully evolved phase (illustrated in Fig.

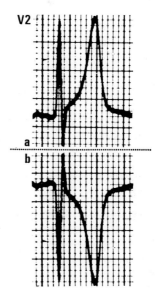

Fig. 40. (a) Enlargement of lead V2 of Fig. 39 showing tall R wave and tall symmetrical T wave. (b) Mirror-image of lead V2 showing deep broad 'Q wave' and deep symmetrical 'T wave'.

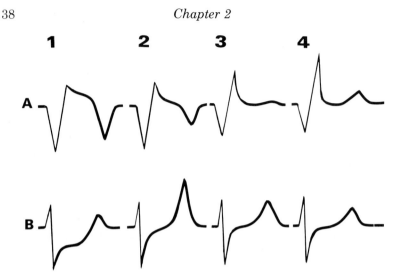

Fig. 41. Diagrams illustrating the resolution of myocardial infarction. (A) Lead orientated to the injured surface. (B) Lead orientated to the uninjured surface.

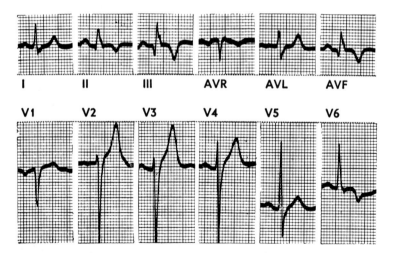

Fig. 42. Electrocardiogram showing the features of recent inferolateral myocardial infarction. Note the Q wave, coved S-T segment and acutely inverted T wave in Standard leads II and III, and lead AVF; lead V6 shows a coved S-T segment with inverted T wave indicating lateral extension of the infarct. The coved S-T segments are not elevated and tall symmetrical T waves are present in leads V2 to V4 indicating that the infarct is probably about 2 weeks old.

41). During the few weeks after the fully evolved phase, there is a gradual return of the elevated S-T segments to the baseline. Concomitantly, *tall symmetrical T waves* appear in leads orientated to the *uninjured surface* (illustrated by Diagram 2 of Fig. 41; and Fig. 42). The abnormal T waves gradually return to a normal or near-normal configuration (illustrated by Diagram 3 of Fig. 41). The pattern then stabilizes into a residual state where the only evidence of a previous myocardial infarction may be an abnormal Q wave in leads orientated to the infarct scar (illustrated by Diagram 4 of Fig. 41; and Fig. 43). It must be emphasized, however, that although the electrocardiographic features of ischaemia and injury may regress, the S-T segment and T wave will still frequently reflect the stigmata of coronary insufficiency, e.g. horizontality of the S-T segment, symmetry of the T wave (see page 45).

It is clear that the acuteness of a myocardial infarction is diagnosed electrocardiographically primarily by the behaviour of the S-T segment and the T wave. Thus:

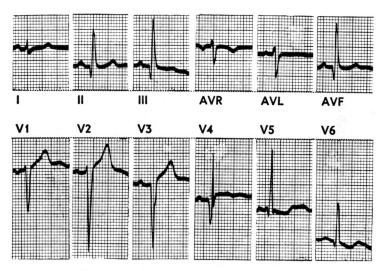

Fig. 43. Electrocardiogram showing the features of old inferior and anterolateral myocardial infarctions. Pathological Q waves are present in Standard leads II and III, and lead AVF (inferior infarction), and leads V4 to V6 (anterolateral infarction). The Q waves are not associated with coved and elevated S-T segments, or acutely inverted T waves, thus indicating old infarction. Note the presence of a QS complex in lead V3 and a significant pathological Q wave in lead V4, which diminishes in depth from leads V4 to V6, reflecting an anterolateral infarct. Note, too, the 'mirror-image correction mark' shape of the S-T segments in leads V5 and V6 due to digitalis effect.

ACUTE INFARCTION

Hyperacute phase

> Slope-elevation of the S-T segment
> Tall widened T wave
> Increased ventricular activation time

Fully evolved phase

> Pathological Q wave
> Coved and elevated S-T segment
> Inverted symmetrical T wave

OLD INFARCTION

> Pathological Q wave
> S-T segments and T waves which may be normal, equivocal or
> diagnostic of coronary insufficiency.

VENTRICULAR ANEURYSM

Note: The persistence of the typical pattern of the fully evolved phase
of myocardial infarction—Q wave, raised S-T segment and inverted T
wave—for 3 months or longer after the acute attack, suggests the
development of a **ventricular aneurysm.** See also section 'Northwest' Axis in Chapter 7, page 121.

EVALUATION OF Q WAVE SIGNIFICANCE IN MYOCARDIAL INFARCTION

The following factors must be taken into consideration in the
assessment of a Q wave with significance to myocardial infarction:

(a) The specific leads in which the Q waves appear.
(b) The number of leads in which the Q waves appear.
(c) The width and depth of the Q wave.
(d) The presence of associated bundle branch block.
(e) Collateral electrocardiographic evidence of myocardial infarction or coronary insufficiency.

Normal Q waves

Small q waves are normally present with normal intraventricular conduction in (*a*) the left precordial leads, lead AVL and Standard lead I with a horizontal heart position or left axis deviation; (*b*) in Standard leads II, III and lead AVF with a vertical heart position or right axis deviation. These small q waves are but a reflection of normal septal activation.

Deep wide Q waves or QS complexes are normally present in lead AVR, and may possibly also be present in lead V1. This is due to the fact that the positive poles of these leads are orientated towards the cavity or the basal regions of the heart, so that the activation process moves away from these leads (see page 122).

Pathological Q waves

Pathological Q waves have the following characteristics:

(*a*) The Q wave is **wide**, 0.04 sec in duration or longer.

(*b*) The Q wave is **deep**, usually greater than 4 mm in depth.

(*c*) The Q wave is usually associated with a **substantial loss in the height of the ensuring R wave**. A rough but not invariably accurate guide is a Q wave whose depth is more than 25 per cent of the height of the ensuing R wave.

(*d*) The aforementioned pathological Q wave characteristics must appear in leads which do not normally have deep and wide Q waves, i.e. they have no significance of infarction when they appear in leads AVR and possibly lead V1 (see above).

(*e*) **Pathological Q waves are usually present in several leads**, for example with inferior infarction, Q waves will be present in Standard leads II, III and lead AVF; with anterolateral infarction, pathological Q waves will be present in Standard lead AVL and the lateral precordial leads—leads V5 and V6.

Q waves and bundle branch block

In the presence of *right bundle branch block*, q or Q waves generally have the same significance as when they are associated with normal intraventricular conduction, since the advent of right bundle branch block does not materially affect the initial vector (see page 75).

In the presence of *left bundle branch block*, the normal septal q waves disappear from leads orientated to the left ventricle—usually leads V5 and V6. Thus, in the presence of left bundle branch block, the manifestation in these leads of any small initial q wave—no matter how small—is therefore pathological, and usually signifies myocardial infarction; an infarction that usually involves the interventricular septum.

Furthermore, in uncomplicated left bundle branch block, Q waves or QS complexes which resemble the pathological Q waves of myocardial infarction may appear in leads orientated to the right ventricle—particularly lead V1. This is an effect of the left bundle branch block and does not signify infarction.

THE SIGNIFICANCE OF A Q WAVE IN STANDARD LEAD III

A Q wave in Standard lead III (associated with a normal S-T segment and T wave) may be the result of an **old** inferior infarction. However, a Q wave in this lead may frequently be present normally, and it may also occur in pathological conditions other than myocardial infarction, e.g. in acute pulmonary embolism and left posterior hemiblock. Thus, the criteria for a Q wave in Standard lead III that is suggestive or diagnostic of an old inferior infarction requires further clarification.

A Q wave in Standard lead III is suggestive of an old inferior infarction when the following criteria are satisfied:
1.   The duration of the Q wave must be at least 0.04 sec, i.e. one small square in width.
2.   A Q wave of at least 0.02 sec in duration, i.e. half a small square in width, must be present in lead AVF.
3.   A q or Q wave of any duration must be present in Standard lead II.
4.   The associated R wave in Standard lead III must be at least 5 mm in height, unless the Q wave in that lead is greater than 2.5 mm.
5.   The P wave in Standard lead III must be upright. This is necessary to exclude some forms of A-V nodal rhythm where an inverted P wave associated with a short P–R interval may mimic a Q wave (see Chapter 14).

Note: A negative delta wave in the W-P-W syndrome may also mimic a pathological Q wave (see Chapter 21, Figs. 200 and 201).

A normal q wave in Standard lead III frequently disappears on deep inspiration; this should be a routine procedure when recording Standard lead III.

See also the vectorial concept of Q wave significance in Standard lead III (page 133).

SUBENDOCARDIAL INFARCTION

Electrocardiographic criteria for the diagnosis of pure or dominant subendocardial infarction are not as definitive or clear cut as that of transmural or even epicardial infarction. The diagnosis is thus mainly a clinical-electrocardiographic correlation. The diagnosis may be entertained when (*a*) the clinical and biochemical presentation suggests acute myocardial infarction, and (*b*) the electrocardiogram presents with depressed S-T segments and deeply inverted T waves in the mid and lateral precordial leads as well as in Standard leads I and II; and these abnormal changes persist for several days (Fig. 44).

It is apparent that the aforementioned S-T segment and T wave changes are, in effect, the mirror-image of those associated with the hyperacute early injury phase of transmural or dominantly subepicardial infarction, or the mirror-image of the electrocardiographic manifestations of the variant form of angina pectoris. There is little or no alteration of the QRS complex.

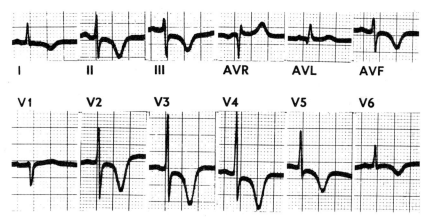

Fig. 44. The electrocardiogram was recorded from a 49-year-old man with typical clinical and biochemical (enzyme) presentation of myocardial infarction. The tracing shows the features commonly associated with acute subendocardial infarction: 1. The S-T segment is depressed with a convex-upward slope in Standard leads I, II and III, and leads AVF and V2 to V6. 2. The T waves are widened and inverted in Standard leads I, II and III, and leads AVF, and V2 to V6. The T wave axis is directed posteriorly and at −110° on the frontal plane hexaxial reference system. *Note*: 1. The S-T segment depression with inverted T wave, best seen in Standard leads II and III, leads AVF and V2 to V5, is the mirror-image of classic electrocardiographic presentation of the hyperacute early injury phase of dominant subepicardial infarction of the variant angina pectoris. 2. These features regressed within 10 days.

Subendocardial infarction may also be evident from lateral extension of a transmural infarction when leads reflect a pathological Q wave with a diminution in the magnitude of the ensuing R wave (Diagram C of Fig. 22 and, for example, leads V5 and V6 of Fig. 30).

THE ELECTROCARDIOGRAM AS A PROGNOSTIC GUIDE IN MYOCARDIAL INFARCTION

The following electrocardiographic features are usually, but not invariably, associated with a relatively adverse prognosis in acute myocardial infarction:

1. Extensive infarction: The infarction pattern is seen in many leads, e.g. (*a*) *extensive* anterior infarction—the infarction pattern is seen in leads V1 to V6, as well as in lead AVL and Standard lead 1; (*b*) inferolateral infarction with true posterior extension.

2. Multiple infarctions: Acute infarction associated with evidence of pre-existing old infarctions, e.g. acute anterior infarction combined with evidence of old inferior infarction.

3. Bundle branch blocks: The development of bundle branch connotes an adverse prognosis; left bundle branch block is a more adverse prognostic sign than right bundle branch block.

4. Ectopic ventricular rhythms: The following ectopic ventricular rhythms are listed in order of increasing prognostic adversity: frequently unifocal ventricular extrasystoles; unifocal ventricular extrasystoles in bigeminal rhythm; unifocal ventricular extrasystoles in pairs; multifocal ventricular extrasystoles; ventricular tachycardia (see also Fig. 165 and page 187). The manifestation of ventricular extrasystoles with a very short coupling interval—the **'R on T' phenomenon** is particularly ominous (see page 188).

5. Atrioventricular block: The development of atrioventricular block always worsens the prognosis; the higher the degree of block, the more adverse the prognosis (Cohen, Doctor & Pick, 1958[3]). In patients who survive the initial episode, the long-term prognosis is not affected by the persistence of atrioventricular block.

6. Anterior wall infarction: An anterior wall myocardial infarction is usually associated with a more adverse prognosis than inferior wall myocardial infarction.

CORONARY INSUFFICIENCY

Transient myocardial injury and ischaemia. Angina pectoris. The 'minor' signs of coronary artery disease

Coronary artery disease may be reflected by changes in the QRS complex, S-T segment, T wave and the U wave. These changes may be present at rest or they may be precipitated by methods which induce transient myocardial injury and ischaemia, e.g. exercise.

THE ELECTROCARDIOGRAPHIC EFFECTS OF CORONARY INSUFFICIENCY

The QRS deflection represents the activation or depolarization process of the ventricles; the S-T segment and T wave represent the recovery or repolarization process of the ventricles. The effects of coronary insufficiency may be reflected in both processes and in their relationship to each other. The earliest changes, however, are usually evident in repolarization, i.e. in the S-T segment, the T wave and the U wave. As a rule, changes in depolarization tend to be permanent, whereas changes in repolarization tend, at least initially, to be temporary or evanescent.

1. The effects on the QRS complex

Coronary insufficiency may cause **bundle branch block,** particularly left bundle branch block (see Chapter 3), and **significant left axis deviation** (see Chapter 7).

2. The effects on the S-T segment

Coronary insufficiency may **alter the shape** and **depress** the S-T segment. It may, on occasion, also present with transient *elevation* of the S-T segment as a manifestation of the variant form of angina pectoris—Prinzmental's Angina.

THE EFFECT ON THE SHAPE OF THE S-T SEGMENT

Horizontality of the S-T segment

Normally, the S-T segment merges smoothly, gradually and imperceptibly with the ascending limb of the T wave so that a separation

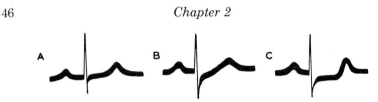

Fig. 45. Diagrammatic illustration showing (A) normal QRST complex, (B) junctional S-T segment depression, (C) plane S-T segment depression.

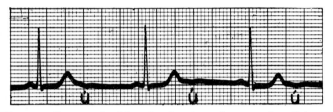

Fig. 46. Electrocardiogram—lead V5—showing signs of coronary insufficiency. There is horizontality of the S-T segment, a sharp-angled ST-T junction and inverted U wave.

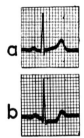

Fig. 47. Electrocardiogram—lead V5. (a) Before exercise, showing normal QRST complex. Note how the S-T segment moves smoothly and imperceptibly with the T wave. (b) After exercise, showing signs of coronary insufficiency, viz. plane depression of the S-T segment with sharp-angled ST-T junction.

between the two is difficult or impossible to define (A in Fig. 45; a in Fig. 47).

One of the earliest signs of coronary insufficiency is an alteration in the shape of the S-T segment, resulting in a **sharp-angled ST-T junction** (Figs. 46, 47 and 49E). The effect is an appearance of **horizontality** of the S-T segment.

DEPRESSION OF THE S-T SEGMENT

A further stage in the evolution of this effect is **depression of the S-T segment**—the depression of coronary insufficiency S-T segment gives the appearance of **plane depression** (Figs. 45C; 47, 48, 60 and

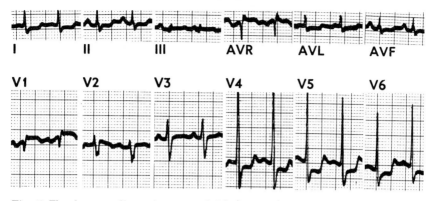

Fig. 48. The electrocardiogram was recorded during an attack of angina pectoris and shows the following: A. Sinus tachycardia. The rate is 125 beats per minute. B. Acute subendocardial injury. This is reflected by the marked plane depression of the S-T segments with sharp angled ST-T junction in leads V4 to V6, Standard leads I and II, and lead AVL. Lead AVR shows reciprocal elevation of the S-T segment. The mean manifest frontal plane S-T segment vector is directed at − 150°.

Comment: The subendocardial injury is dominantly apical, as evidenced by the S-T segment depression in the left lateral leads, and the typical S-T segment vector deviation to − 150°. This reflects the classic localization usually associated with angina pectoris.

61; see below). The S-T segment may also have a **sagging depression** (Fig. 49).

The mechanism of S-T segment depression

Transient myocardial ischaemia, as manifested clinically by the classic form of angina pectoris, results in transient subendocardial injury to the subendocardial apical region of the left ventricle. The injured surface faces the left ventricular cavity (Fig. 50).

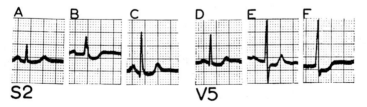

Fig. 49. Electrocardiograms—Standard lead II and lead V5—illustrating various forms of S-T segment depression. Examples A, B, C, D and F illustrate *sagging depression*. Example E illustrates plane depression; note the sharp-angled ST-T junction.

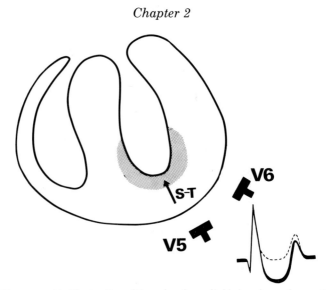

Fig. 50. Diagrammatic illustration of the subendocardial injury in angina pectoris. The transient injury results in an S-T segment shift towards the injured surface, i.e. towards the left ventricular cavity and away from leads V5 and V6; thereby resulting in S-T segment depression in these leads.

On the basis of the principles discussed earlier in this chapter, the S-T segment is deviated to the surface of injury. Thus, a lead orientated to the injured surface—in this case the left ventricular cavity—e.g. lead AVR, will reflect the pattern of injury, a raised S-T segment. Leads facing the external surface—mainly leads V5 and V6—will reflect reciprocal S-T segment depression. These changes are discussed in greater detail with reference to the exercise test (see below and Fig. 50).

Junctional S-T segment depression

Junctional S-T segment depression refers to depression of the *proximal* part of the S-T segment, viz. its junction with the QRS complex. While the proximal part of the S-T segment is depressed, the distal part still rises to merge smoothly and imperceptibly with the T wave.

Junctional S-T segment depression is frequently a physiological phenomenon, and may indeed be an expression of a normal and healthy heart. It is usually due to the depressing effect of the P-Ta segment deflection representing atrial repolarization; and the Ta or Tp wave, the atrial T wave—the atrial repolarization wave—which is

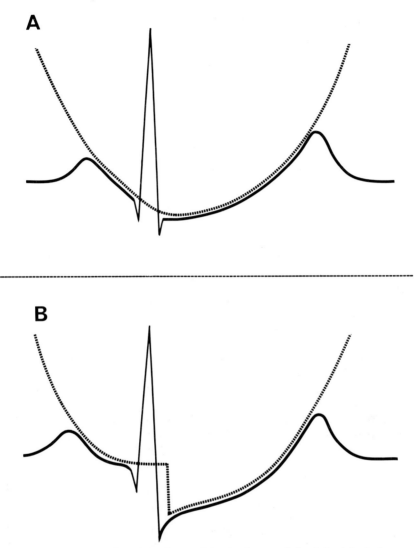

Fig. 51. Diagrams illustrating: (A) the normal unbroken parabola of physiological junctional S-T segment depression, and (B) the broken parabola of abnormal junctional S-T segment depression.

normally *opposite in direction to the P wave.* Junctional S-T segment depression may also, at times (though rarely), be an expression of coronary insufficiency. The significance of junctional S-T segment depression may thus be difficult to evaluate.

A possible method for distinguishing between the junctional

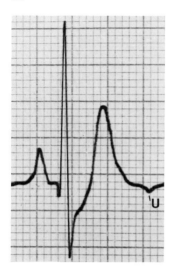

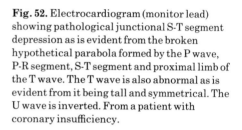

Fig. 52. Electrocardiogram (monitor lead) showing pathological junctional S-T segment depression as is evident from the broken hypothetical parabola formed by the P wave, P-R segment, S-T segment and proximal limb of the T wave. The T wave is also abnormal as is evident from it being tall and symmetrical. The U wave is inverted. From a patient with coronary insufficiency.

depression of physiological origin and pathological origin is the use of a hypothetical parabola, joining the P-R segment, S-T segment and proximal limb of the T wave (Fig. 51; Schamroth, 1975[25]). An unbroken, parabola indicates, in all probability, a normal physiological response. A broken parabola probably indicates true pathological S-T segment depression and constitutes a pointer to the presence of coronary insufficiency (Fig. 52). It must, however, be emphasized that the diagnosis of coronary insufficiency should rarely, if ever, be based solely on the presence of junctional S-T segment depression.

CLASSIC ANGINA PECTORIS

Classic angina pectoris—Heberden's angina—is reflected electrocardiographically by depression of the S-T segment in leads V5 and V6. It may also manifest in Standard lead I or Standard lead II. This is the expression of transient subendocardial injury.

THE VARIANT FORM OF ANGINA PECTORIS

(Synonyms: Prinzmetal's Angina, Atypical Angina)

As noted above (page 47), the classic form of angina pectoris is the expression of transient sub*endo*cardial injury. In contrast to this, the variant form of angina pectoris is due to transient sub*epi*cardial injury. The condition thus manifests characteristically with transient elevation of the S-T segments in leads orientated to the injured surface (see below).

Attention was first focused on this form of angina pectoris by Prinzmetal and his associates (1959),[22] although occasional reports had appeared previously.[10] The condition is not uncommon but has been poorly documented. It is receiving increasing attention,[5] and is now very topical (Maseri and associates, 1975).[16, 17]

ELECTROCARDIOGRAPHIC MANIFESTATIONS

The following electrocardiographic features appear in leads orientated to the injured surface—usually leads V4 to V6 (Figs. 53, 54 and 178):

1. Slope-elevation of the S-T segment.
2. Tall and widened T wave.
3. Increased ventricular activation time.

These three manifestations constitute the classic presentation of the variant form of angina pectoris, a presentation which is, in effect, the same as that of the hyperacute phase of myocardial infarction. In the case of the variant angina pectoris, however, the manifestation is very transient, lasting from a few to about 20 minutes, whereas in the

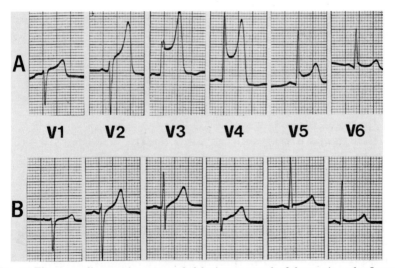

Fig. 53. Electrocardiogram A was recorded during an attack of chest pain and reflects the features of the variant form—Prinzmetal's—angina pectoris. Note the elevated S-T segments and tall T waves in leads V2 to V5. Electrocardiogram B was recorded a few minutes later following the cessation of the chest pain.

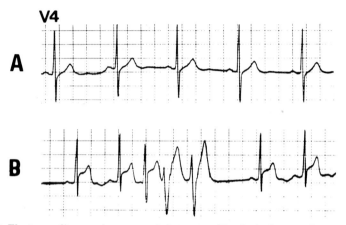

Fig. 54. Electrocardiogram A was recorded at rest and is relatively normal. Electrocardiogram B was recorded after effort and shows the manifestations of the variant form of angina pectoris: increased amplitude of the R wave, diminished amplitude of the S wave slope-elevation of the S-T segments, increased amplitude of the T waves, inverted U waves and ventricular extrasystoles.

hyperacute phase of myocardial infarction, the condition lasts for hours or even days. These electrocardiographic features are described in greater detail in the section on the hyperacute phase of myocardial infarction (page 24 and Diagram B of Fig. 25).

ADDITIONAL FEATURES

4.   Increase in the amplitude of the R wave (Figs. 53 and 54).
5.   Diminution in the depth of the S wave of an RS complex (Figs. 53 and 54).
6.   Transient left anterior hemiblock.[2, 24]
7.   Inversion of the U wave[26] (Fig. 54).
8.   Ventricular extrasystoles or even ventricular tachycardia (Fig. 54).
9.   Transient A-V block.

SIGNIFICANCE

The disorder is due to a marked narrowing of a major coronary artery[6, 14, 15, 20, 22] and is most commonly due to a marked spasm of an otherwise normal, near-normal or diseased coronary artery.[7, 35]

The variant form of angina pectoris is usually associated with a grave clinical prognosis. Infarction and/or death not infrequently occurs within one year of the onset.[8, 9, 19, 21, 23, 31]

3. The effects on the T wave

The T wave is the most unstable component of the electrocardio-graphic recording. Changes of this deflection may occur with ‚hyperventilation, heavy meals, anxiety, smoking, drinking iced water, changes in body position and decrease in blood pressure. Variations also occur with race and age. They are found so frequently as normal variants that when they occur as isolated phenomena their diagnostic import is uncertain.

Despite this, there are certain T wave changes that are frequently suggestive of coronary insufficiency. The normal T wave is asymmetrical. The T wave associated with coronary insufficiency has **symmetrical limbs** and **a sharp-pointed, arrowhead vertex** or **nadir** (Fig. 55a). When the symmetrical, sharply pointed arrowhead T wave is inverted the associated S-T segment usually shows an upward convexity. The abnormal T wave associated with left ventricular 'strain' or digitalis effect usually has asymmetrical limbs with a relatively blunt vertex or nadir (Fig 55b and c).

Coronary insufficiency is also suggested when T waves in many leads are low or inverted.

Occasionally the **T wave becomes taller (as well as pointed and symmetrical)** with coronary insufficiency (Figs. 57 and 59). If, following exercise, the height of the T wave in lead V4 is 5 mm or more than the resting value, coronary insufficiency should be suspected (Lepeschkin & Surawics, 1958).[11]

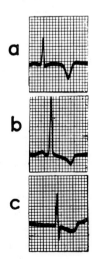

Fig. 55. Electrocardiograms (all of lead V5) showing the S-T segment and T waves changes of: (a) coronary insufficiency: symmetrical, sharply pointed arrowhead inverted T wave with upward convexity of the S-T segment. (b) the 'strain' pattern usually associated with ventricular hypertrophy: asymmetrical T wave with blunt nadir. (c) digitalis effect: asymmetrical T wave with S-T segment and T wave reflecting the mirror-image of a correction mark.

THE QRS:T RELATIONSHIP

In the presence of a dominantly positive QRS deflection in Standard lead I, frank inversion of the T wave in that lead is usually abnormal. Furthermore, in the presence of a dominantly positive QRS deflection in Standard lead I, a **T wave in Standard lead I that is lower than a T wave in Standard lead III** is also frequently abnormal (Fig. 56). The T wave eventually becomes frankly inverted in Standard lead I and very dominantly upright in Standard lead III (Fig. 57). This empirical manifestation is the expression of a wide frontal plane QRS-T angle, i.e. a wide spread between the mean frontal plane QRS and T wave forces (see page 124).

A wide spread between the mean QRS and T wave forces may also be reflected by the precordial leads, i.e. the horizontal plane leads (see page 127 and Fig. 122). Empirically, this will result in a **T wave that is taller in lead V1 than in lead V6,** associated with a QRS complex that is dominant and upright in lead V6 (Fig. 57). This finding is suggestive of coronary insufficiency and may be one of its earliest signs (Weyn & Marriott, 1962[34]). Further progression results in frank inversion of the T wave in lead V6 (Fig. 58).

4. The effects on the U wave

The U wave is a small rounded deflection occurring just after the T

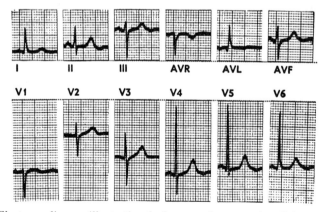

Fig. 56. Electrocardiogram illustrating the features of coronary insufficiency. *Note:* (*a*) the T wave in Standard lead I is lower than the T wave in Standard lead III: the expression of a wide QRS-T angle of 70°—the frontal plane QRS axis is directed at − 10°, the frontal plane T wave axis is directed at + 60°; (*b*) inversion of the U wave in Standard leads II and III, lead AVF, and leads V4 to V6; (*c*) rather horizontal S-T segments in Standard lead II and lead V6.

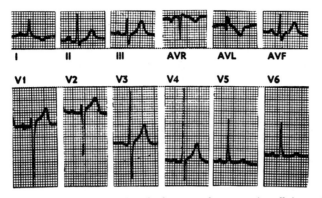

Fig. 57. Electrocardiogram illustrating the features of coronary insufficiency. Note (*a*) inversion of the T wave in Standard lead I, associated with a tall dominant T wave in Standard lead III; (*b*) the T wave in lead V1 is taller than the T wave in lead V6.

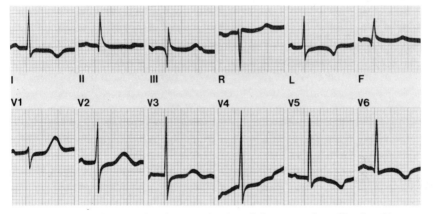

Fig. 58. Electrocardiogram showing coronary insufficiency as reflected by the wide frontal and horizontal plane QRS-T angles. The T wave vector is directed to the right—away from the ischaemic left ventricle. Thus, the QRS axis is directed at + 30°. The T wave axis is directed at + 150°. The QRS-T angle is 120°. This is also reflected in the horizontal plane where the T waves are inverted in the left precordial leads—V5 and V6—and upright in the right precordial leads—V1 to V3, thereby connoting a rightward deviation of the horizontal plane T wave axis—away from the ischaemic left ventricle. The coronary insufficiency is also reflected by the symmetry of the inverted T waves.

wave (Figs. 64 and 241). It is best seen in the precordial leads reflecting the transition zone—usually V2 to V4. It is normally in the same direction as the T wave. The deflection may be so small as to make accurate recognition difficult; and, in the presence of a

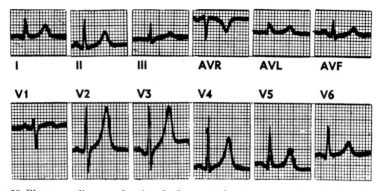

Fig. 59. Electrocardiogram showing the features of acute coronary insufficiency. Note the tall, peaked symmetrical arrowhead T waves in leads V2 to V6 and in Standard leads I and II.

tachycardia, the U wave may be superimposed on the following P wave making recognition impossible (half-minute tracing in Fig. 60).

An inverted U wave, i.e. a U wave that is opposite in direction to the T wave, is diagnostic of cardiac disease, especially of coronary artery or hypertensive origin (Fig. 64). When it develops after exercise it always indicates cardiac ischaemia (Figs. 54 and 60).

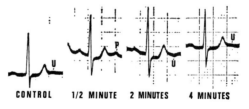

Fig. 60. Electrocardiographic recording during an exercise test. Standard lead I. *Note*: Positive U wave in the control tracing and an inverted U wave in the 2-minute tracing; superimposition of the P wave on the U wave during the tachycardia of the half-minute tracing; 1.25 mm *plane* depression of the S-T segment with *sharp-angled ST-T junction* in the half-minute and 2-minute tracings; the smooth transition of the ST-T junction in the control tracing; the downward slope of the P-R segment in the half-minute tracing. There is also a prolonged P–R interval in the control and 4-minute tracings.

Comment: the S-T segment depression, plane configuration of the S-T segment with sharp-angled ST-T junction and inverted U wave makes this test definitely positive and diagnostic of coronary insufficiency.

Comment

While many of the aforementioned electrocardiographic signs are indicative, presumptive or suggestive of coronary insufficiency, it must be emphasized that the diagnosis must *not* be based on equivocal or non-pathognomonic signs, e.g. minor T wave changes, isolated T wave changes, or junctional S-T segment depression. And it cannot be stressed too strongly that clinical judgment is paramount and that too much weight must not be placed on an equivocal electrocardiographic change as the sole criterion of coronary insufficiency.

THE EXERCISE TEST

THE PURPOSE OF THE EXERCISE TEST

A good history is usually sufficient to establish the diagnosis of angina pectoris or coronary insufficiency. At times, however, the pain is atypical and the history doubtful; objective confirmation of the diagnosis then becomes desirable. In such cases, the electrocardiographic changes seen in response to exercise may provide this confirmatory evidence, since the object of the test is to increase the demand for coronary blood flow where an inadequate flow is suspected.

THE PERFORMANCE OF THE EXERCISE TEST

The exercise test can be performed according to a standardized or a non-standardized method.

The standardized method

Master and his associates (1942)[18] standardized the test according to sex, weight and age. Using these parameters, tables were constructed based on the return of blood pressure and pulse rate to normal within 2 minutes. The exercise is performed on a special standardized two-step apparatus and the patient is required to do a certain number of ascents and descents in $1\frac{1}{2}$ minutes.

The principles may well be questioned, for it has not been shown that coronary artery disease, once present, runs a course which is more severe in the female; nor has it been shown that electrocardiographic changes following exercise parallel those of pulse rate and blood pressure. Furthermore, although coronary artery disease is usually more prevalent and more marked in the older age groups, it may be severe in a woman of 40 years and not at all evident in a man of 80 years.

In addition, other factors, such as emotion and training, may influence the outcome of the test and will affect any attempt to standardize it.

Nevertheless, although the validity of the exercise test as described by Master may be questioned, it should be stated that the Master two-step test is recognized in many centres and is commonly used as a routine procedure in many electrocardiographic laboratories. Provided its limitations are appreciated, it may serve a purpose as a comparative standard, e.g. (i) as a standard for insurance evaluation; (ii) as a uniform screening test in the medical examination of military and aviation personnel; (iii) as a possible research standard. This method is now being increasingly replaced by exercise ergometry—treadmill or bicycle ergometry.

The non-standard method

Scherf recommended originally (1935)[27] and later (1960),[29] that the amount of exercise the patient is required to perform be adapted to the needs of the particular individual. This is particularly appropriate to consulting room practice. The patient is subjected to approximately the exertion that has been known, or assessed, to bring on an attack of angina pectoris. This does not mean that the patient is exercised indiscriminately until such time as he develops pain. If, for example, the patient has pain after only the slightest exertion, he may be asked to do a few knee-bends or sit up and down a few times; whereas a patient who has pain only after severe exertion may be asked to climb several flights of stairs rapidly.

If no changes are noted, and if the patient's condition warrants it, the exercise test may be repeated after a suitable interval (usually 1 hour) with a cautious increase in the amount of exercise.

The following procedures are thus recommended in the performance of the exercise test:

1. The *patient must not be in pain.* The history and physical examination must not suggest an impending myocardial infarction or acute pulmonary embolism. The patient must not be in congestive cardiac failure.

2. An electrocardiogram is recorded at rest and must be normal or at most equivocal in respect of coronary artery disease. There must be *no tachycardia.*

3.   The test is preferably performed *before a meal*, since physiological electrocardiographic variants are more likely to occur after a meal. If the patient relates a history of angina pectoris after meals, the test should then be performed before a meal and, if negative, repeated after a meal.

4.   The exercise test is performed according to the non-standardized method.

5.   If pain, substernal discomfort, a feeling of faintness or pallor develop during the performance of the test, the exercise is stopped immediately. Exercise to the point of pain is hazardous and unjustifiable. *The attendance of a physician is mandatory.*

6.   The electrocardiogram is recorded immediately after the exercise and at 2-minute intervals for 6 minutes, or until such time as it returns to the resting configuration.

7.   The electrocardiographic changes should be observed in at least one precordial lead and one extremity or bipolar lead. S-T segment changes are usually best seen in leads with the tallest R waves—commonly leads V5 and V6, and Standard lead II; this is due to the fact that these leads are usually orientated towards the main muscle mass of the ventricles (see page 124 and Figs. 118 and 119). T wave changes that occur in Standard lead I are usually the most significant of those seen in the Standard leads when the QRS axis is directed to the region of 0°. T wave changes that occur in Standard lead II are usually the most significant of those seen in the Standard leads when the QRS axis is directed to +60°.

8.   The test must *not* be performed if the patient is reluctant or unco-operative.

THE INTERPRETATION OF THE EXERCISE TEST

Certain electrocardiographic changes which follow exercise are always pathological; others, however, can only be regarded as normal physiological variants. The transition between normal and abnormal, however, may be extremely difficult, if not impossible, to define; and there is a considerable degree of overlap between the two. Since it is never possible to rule out false negative tests, i.e. a normal electrocardiogram does not necessarily exclude coronary artery disease, it is best to establish stringent criteria of major abnormality in order to avoid labelling borderline physiological variants as abnormal. Less stringent criteria are used for insurance purposes and the screening of military and aviation personnel, and as possible pointers to the presence of coronary artery disease.

The electrocardiographic changes which follow exercise may affect all components of the record—the P wave, the P-R segment, the QRS complex, the S-T segment, the T wave and the U wave; in addition, abnormal rhythms may occur. These changes are summarized in Table 2. Most of the significant changes have already been described above in the section titled 'The Electrocardiographic Effects of Coronary Insufficiency'; it must be stressed that these changes have the same significance when precipitated by exercise as when present in the 'resting' or control tracing.

CHANGES AFFECTING THE P WAVE (Table 2)

Following exercise there is a tendency for *right axis deviation of the P wave*, so that the P waves tend to become taller in Standard leads II and III. This is a normal physiological variant (Fig. 60).

CHANGES AFFECTING THE P-R SEGMENT (Table 2)

The *P-R interval normally shortens with exercise* (Fig. 60).

The effect on the Tp wave

Atrial depolarization is normally followed by atrial repolarization, i.e. as a T wave follows the QRS complex, so a corresponding 'T' wave normally follows the P wave. This atrial T wave is known as the Ta or Tp wave and is normally opposite in direction to the P wave. It is usually masked by the ensuing QRST deflection and is therefore best seen following isolated P waves such as occurs during A-V block.

Following exercise, the Tp deflection normally becomes more pronounced in those leads where the P wave becomes taller (see above), and may cause the P-R segment to have a downward slope (Fig. 60, half-minute and 2-minute tracings). Since this Tp deflection is superimposed upon the proximal part of the S-T junction. It may cause junctional depression of the S-T segment, thus producing false positive S-T segment depression.

CHANGES AFFECTING THE QRS COMPLEX

See Table 2; and also the section above, titled 'The Electrocardiographic Effects of Coronary Insufficiency'.

Component of ECG	Abnormal	Usually abnormal	Physiological or diagnostically uncertain
P wave			Some rightward deviation (taller in Standard leads II and III)
P-R segment ...			Downward slope
QRS complex ...	Left bundle branch block	Right bundle branch block Left axis deviation	Some rightward deviation
S-T segment ...	Depression of 2 mm or more in the precordial leads	Depression of 0.75–2 mm in the precordial leads Any degree of plane or sagging depression	Some forms of junctional depression
	Depression of 1.5 mm or more in the extremity leads	'Horizontality' Sharp-angled ST-T junction Some forms of junctional depression	
T wave		Inversion in Standard lead I and leads V5 and V6 T in Standard lead I lower than T in Standard lead III Increase in height by 5 mm or more in lead V4 Symmetrical T waves—upright or inverted	
U wave	Inversion		
Ventricular extrasystoles...	Multifocal	Unifocal: In 'showers' In bigeminal rhythm In a patient over 40 years	Isolated unifocal
	Post-extrasystolic T wave change Post-extrasystolic U wave change		

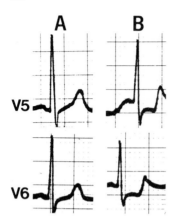

Fig. 61. Electrocardiogram (leads V5 and V6). A = recorded at rest. B = recorded immediately after effort showing plane S-T segment depression.

Following exercise there is a *normal tendency for some rightward deviation* of the QRS axis.

The development of abnormal widening of the QRS complex is regarded as an abnormal test. The appearance of **left bundle branch block** after exercise is likewise abnormal. The development of right bundle branch block is usually abnormal but may occasionally occur as a normal variant, especially when it is dependent upon critical rate (see Fig. 220, page 263). The development of left axis deviation after exercise is usually abnormal.

CHANGES AFFECTING THE S-T SEGMENT

See Table 2; see also the section above, titled 'The Electrocardiographic Effects of Coronary Insufficiency'.

Coronary insufficiency causes S-T segment depression. This is best seen in leads with the tallest R waves—usually lead V5 and Standard lead II, or Standard lead I if there is left axis deviation (see page 116).

The degree of depression that is considered definitely abnormal is probably the most disputed point in the interpretation of the exercise test. Figures in excess of 0.5 mm (Master *et al.*, 1942[18]), 0.75 mm (Lepeschkin & Surawics, 1958[11]; Levan, 1945[12]), 1.0 mm (Unterman & de Graff, 1948[33]), 1.5 mm (Biorck, 1946[1]) and 2 mm (Scherf & Schaffer, 1952[30]) depression in the precordial leads V4 and V5 have all been considered as definitely abnormal. The matter is further complicated by the fact that it is at times difficult to judge the position of the baseline as a reference point from which to measure the depression. The depressing effect of the Tp deflection must also be taken into account (see above). The best baseline or isoelectric level to use is the U-P segment, but this is often obscured during the tachycardia which so frequently follows exertion (half-minute recording in Fig. 60). In such cases the baseline is measured from the junction of the P-R segment with QRS complex.

The approach as evaluated by Scherf & Schaffer (1952)[30] is based on the premise that, since it is impossible to eliminate false negative tests, i.e. since a negative result or normal electrocardiogram does not exclude cardiac disease, it becomes imperative to avoid false positive tests, consequent incorrect diagnoses, and possible iatrogenic disease. Thus, Scherf deliberately set extremely stringent criteria to avoid making incorrect diagnoses; so that a positive test should be based on incontestable standards. The test is therefore, in Scherf's evaluation, only considered diagnostically positive when the S-T segment depression is 2 mm or more in the precordial leads and 1.5 mm or more in the extremity leads. Nevertheless, any depression of between 0.75 mm and 2 mm in the precordial leads is usually abnormal (Figs. 48, 60 and 61). Indeed, it is abundantly clear nowadays that even S-T segment horizontality without depression should be viewed with suspicion, and any element of S-T segment depression that is not junctional probably reflects abnormality (see section on 'Junctional S-T Segment Depression', page 48).

CHANGES AFFECTING THE T WAVE

Table 2, and also the section above, titled 'The Electrocardiographic Effects of Coronary Insufficiency'.

CHANGES AFFECTING THE U WAVE

Table 2; and also the section above titled, 'The Electrocardiographic Effects of Coronary Insufficiency'.

CHANGES IN RHYTHM FOLLOWING EXERCISE
(Table 2)

Sinus tachycardia normally follows exercise.

The presence of **multiform ventricular extrasystoles** is diagnostic of cardiac disease. When they develop in response to exercise they constitute a positive test.

Unifocal ventricular extrasystoles may occasionally be found in the normal subject. Nevertheless, their presence after exercise usually means abnormality; especially if they occur in 'showers', if they give rise to short runs of bigeminal rhythm, if they occur in a person over 40 years of age or if they persist for several minutes or longer. Ventricular extrasystoles which are precipitated by exercise and tachycardia are more frequently associated with cardiac disease than those ventricular extrasystoles which are abolished by exercise and tachycardia.

ADDITIONAL FACTORS

THE DURATION OF ECG ABNORMALITIES AFTER EXERCISE

Electrocardiographic changes, particularly S-T segment depression, due to coronary insufficiency tend to last longer than those caused by physiological variants. Although there are exceptions, normal variants or false positive changes usually last less than 2 minutes, whereas pathological or true positive changes commonly last 5 minutes or longer (Lepeschkin & Surawics, 1958[11]).

Horizontality of the S-T segment or, for example, an S-T segment depression of about 0·05 mm in the precordial leads, which is usually, though not definitely, diagnostic of cardiac ischaemia, is considerably strengthened as a criterion of positivity when the change last 5 minutes or longer.

THE EFFECT OF DIGITALIS ON THE EXERCISE TEST

Digitalis may markedly influence the S-T segment (see page 93 and Figs. 55 and 87) and positive tests have been reported in patients taking digitalis, in whom there was no evidence of coronary artery disease (Zwillinger, 1935[36]; Liebow & Feil, 1941[13]). The exercise test cannot, therefore, be interpreted with confidence in the presence of digitalis effect.

HYPERTENSION AND THE EXERCISE TEST

The exercise test should be interpreted with caution when there is associated hypertension with left ventricular hypertrophy and strain, since this may, at times, mimic the effects of coronary insufficiency. Following exercise, a pattern of left ventricular hypertrophy (QRS changes only) may change to one of 'strain'—S-T segment depression with T wave inversion; U wave inversion may also occur. Such T wave change, however, usually manifests with asymmetrical limbs and the vertex is not pointed (see above and Fig. 55b).

RELATIONSHIP OF ELECTROCARDIOGRAPHIC CHANGES TO THE DEVELOPMENT OF PAIN

The appearance of abnormal electrocardiographic changes does not necessarily correlate with that of pain. Although the patient should *not* be exercised to the point of pain by intent, when pain is precipitated as a result of the exercise test it may occur long after the appearance of abnormal changes and may disappear long before such changes have regressed.

POST EXTRASYSTOLIC T AND U WAVE CHANGE

THE 'POOR MAN'S EXERCISE TEST'

Levine has styled the chance finding of an extrasystole with **post-extrasystolic T wage change** in the control tracing as a 'poor man's exercise test', since it reflects immediate evidence of abnormality and obviates the necessity for a further, more expensive, exercise test.

The abnormality consists of a T wave change in the first *sinus* beat following an atrial or ventricular extrasystole (Figs. 62 and 63). The T wave usually becomes inverted, but may become taller than normal. Any change is significant. particularly when the T wave is inverted, symmetrical and arrowhead, in appearance. Similar changes have been observed following blocked atrial extrasystoles (Scherf, 1944[25]) (Fig. 63). Thus, it is not the extrasystole *per se* that causes this change, but rather it is the pause it occasions that evokes the change (Scherf, 1944[28]). It may also manifest after a sudden long pause during atrial fibrillation.

The U wave may also become momentarily inverted following an extrasystole—**post-extrasystolic U wave inversion** (Fig. 64). This manifestation is definitely abnormal.

PERICARDITIS

ACUTE PERICARDITIS

Acute pericarditis injures the epicardial surface of the heart. This

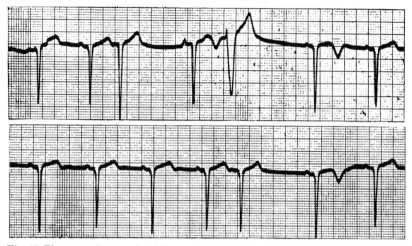

Fig. 62. Electrocardiogram (lead V1, continuous strip) showing post-extrasystolic T wave inversion. The third QRS complex in the upper strip and the fifth QRS complex in the lower strip are conducted atrial extrasystoles; the fifth QRS complex in the upper lip is a ventricular extrasystole. Note the marked inversion and symmetry of the T wave in the normal sinus complex *following* the compensatory pause of each extrasystole.

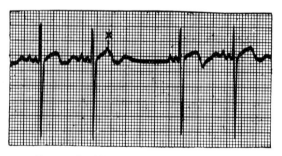

Fig. 63. Electrocardiogram (lead V3) showing a blocked atrial extrasystole with post-extrasystolic T wave inversion. The P wave of the extrasystole—labelled X—is superimposed upon the S-T segment of the second QRST complex. Note the T wave inversion associated with the sinus beat following the extrasystole.

results in a **shell of injured tissue surrounding the heart** (Fig. 65).

This injury is reflected as a raised S-T segment in leads orientated to the affected surface (refer to the Appendix for an explanation of this injury effect). As there is no myocardial ischaemia, the T waves remain upright. This results in a characteristic shape to the S-T segment, viz. it is **raised and concave upwards** (Figs. 65 and 66).

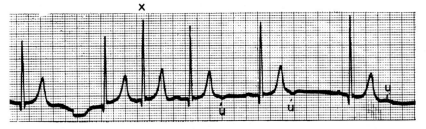

Fig. 64. Electrocardiogram (Standard lead II) showing post-extrasystolic U wave inversion. X represents an atrial extrasystole. Note the U wave inversion in the two sinus beats following the extrasystole.

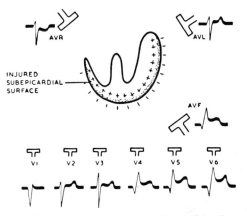

Fig. 65. Diagrammatic illustration of the electrocardiographic effects of acute pericarditis.

This pattern is reflected in all leads facing the injured surface, i.e. most leads except lead AVR which faces the cavity of the heart—the uninjured surface—and thus records a depressed S-T segment, and Standard lead III which usually reflects an equiphasic S-T segment. This is because the S-T segment vector is commonly directed at $+30°$ on the frontal plane hexaxial reference system. The S-T segment vector is thus at right angles to the Standard lead III axis and parallel to the lead AVR axis. It is consequently maximal, but negative, in lead AVR. This contrasts with the S-T segment vector of the hyperacute phase of inferior wall infarction which is directed to the region of $+100°$ and whose configuration may mimic that of acute pericarditis.

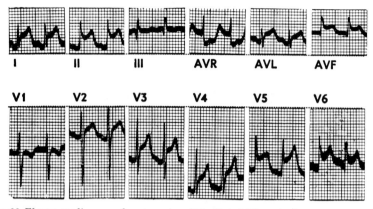

Fig. 66. Electrocardiogram of acute pericarditis. Note (*a*) the raised, concave upward S-T segment in nearly all leads, and (*b*) the sinus tachycardia.

CHRONIC PERICARDITIS. PERICARDIAL EFFUSION. CONSTRICTIVE PERICARDITIS

With resolution of the acute stage of pericarditis, the S-T segments become isoelectric. The development of pericardial effusion or constrictive pericarditis results in **generalized low voltage** and the **T waves become low, isoelectric or inverted** in all leads orientated to the surface of the heart, i.e. most leads excepting lead AVR (Figs. 67 and 68). The low voltage is due to short-circuiting of the electrical impulse through the surrounding fluid or thickened pericardium.

Note. The same electrocardiographic pattern may be due to **myxoedema** or **hypopituitism**. (For other causes of generalized low voltage, see page 298.)

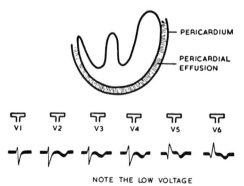

Fig. 67. Diagrammatic illustration of the electrocardiographic effects of pericardial effusion.

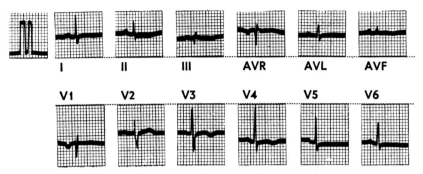

I	II	III	AVR	AVL	AVF

V1	V2	V3	V4	V5	V6

Fig. 68. Electrocardiogram showing the features of pericardial effusion. Note the generalized low voltage and the low to inverted T waves throughout. Standardization is correct, i.e. one millivolt causes a deflection of 1 cm.

SUMMARY

Acute pericarditis

Normal voltage.
Raised, concave upward S-T segments in leads orientated to the heart surface.

Chronic pericarditis

Generalized low voltage.
Low to inverted T waves in leads orientated to the heart surface.

REFERENCES

1 BIORCK B. (1946) Anoxemia and exercise tests in the diagnosis of coronary diseases. *Amer. Heart J.* **32,** 689.
2 BOBBA P., VECCHIO C., DI GUGLIELMO L., SALERNO J., CASARI A. & MONTEMARTINI C. (1972) Exercise-induced RS-T elevation. Electrographic and angiographic observations. *Cardiology* **57,** 162.
3 COHEN D. B., DOCTOR, LE ROY & PICK A. (1958) The significance of atrioventricular block complicating acute myocardial infarction. *Amer. Heart J.* **2,** 215.
4 DUNN W. J., EDWARDS J. E. & PRUITT R. D. (1956) The electrocardiogram in infarction of the lateral wall of the left ventricle. *Circulation* **14,** 540.
5 EDITORIAL (1971) Atypical angina. *Brit. Med. J.* **1,** 62.
6 FORTUIN N. J. & FRIESINGER G. C. (1970) Exercise-induced S-T segment elevation. Clinical, electrocardiographic and arteriographic studies in twelve patients. *Amer. J. Med.* **49,** 459.
7 GIANELLY R., MAGLER F. & HARRISON D. C. (1968) Prinzmetal's variant angina with only slight coronary atherosclerosis. *Calif. Med.* **108,** 129.

8 HARDEL M., BAJOLET A., GUERIN R., ELAERTS J. & GERARD J. (1969) Angor de Prinzmetal. A propos d'un cas complique d'infarctus du myocarde. *Arch. Mal. Coer* **62,** 1267.

9 JOUVE A., GUIRAN J. B., VIALLET H., GRAS A., BLANC M., ARNOUX M., ROUVIER M. & BRUNEL J. C. (1969) Les modifications electrocardiographiques au cours des crises d'angor spontane. A propos de la forme decrite par Prinzmetal. *Arch. Mal. Coeur* **62,** 331.

10 KROOF I. G., JAFFE H. L. & MASTER A.M. (1949) The significance of RS-T elevation in acute coronary insufficiency. *Bull NY Acad. Med.* **25,** 465.

11 LEPESCHKIN E. & SURAWICS B. (1958) Characteristics of true-positive and false-positive results of electrocardiographic Master two-step exercise tests. *New Engl. J. Med.* **258,** 511.

12 LEVAN J. B. (1945) Simple exertional electrocardiography as an aid in diagnosis of coronary insufficiency. *War Med.* **7,** 353.

13 LIEBOW I. M. & FEIL H. (1941) Digitalis and normal work electrocardiogram. *Amer. Heart J.* **22,** 683.

14 MACALPIN R. (1970) Variant angina pectoris (letter). *New Engl. J. Med.* **282,** 1491.

15 MACALPIN R. N. & KATTUS A. A. (1967) Angina pectoris at rest with preservation of exercise capacity—angina inversa. *Circulation* **35–36** (Supp. II), 176 (Abstr.).

16 MASERI A., MIMMO R. & CHIERCHIA S. (1975) Coronary artery spasm as a cause of acute ischemia in patients. Hemodynamic and angiographic documentation. *Clin. Res.* **23,** 195A.

17 MASERI A., MIMMO R. CHIERCHIA S. (1975) Coronary artery spasm as a cause of acute myocardial ischemia in man. *Chest* **68,** 625.

18 MASTER A. M., FRIEDMAN R. & DACK S. (1942) The electrocardiogram after standard exercise as a functional test of the heart. *Amer. Heart J.* **24,** 777.

19 POGGI L., BORY M., PINAS E., D'JOUNO J., DJIANE P., FRANCOIS G., SERRADIMIGNI A. & AUDIER M. (1969) L'enregistrement electrographique continu dans l'angor de Prinzmetal. *Arch. Mal. Coeur* **62,** 1241.

20 PRINZMETAL M., EKMEKCI A., KENNAMER R., KWOCZYNSKI J. K., SHUBIN H. & TOYOSHIMA H. (1960) Variant form of angina pectoris; previous undelineated syndrome. *JAMA* **1,** 794.

21 PRINZMETAL M., EKMEKCI A., TOYOSHIMA H. & KWOCZYNSKI J. K. (1959) Angina pectoris. III. Demonstration of a chemical origin of S-T deviation in classic angina pectoris, its variant form, early myocardial infarction, and some non-cardiac conditions. *Amer. J. Cardiol.* **3,** 276.

22 PRINZMETAL M., KENNAMER R., MERLISS R., WADA T. & BOR N. (1959) Angina pectoris. I. A variant form of angina pectoris. *Amer. J. Med.* **27,** 374.

23 ROBINSON H. S. (1965) Prinzmetal's variant of angina pectoris. *Amer. Heart J.* **70,** 797.

24 RUSER H. R. (1970) Prinzmetalische angina pectoris. *Ztschr. Kreislaufforsch.* **9,** 849.

25 SCHAMROTH L. (1975) *The Electrocardiology of Coronary Artery Disease,* p. 160. Blackwell Scientific Publications, Oxford, England.

26 SCHAMROTH L. & LEVENSTEIN J. (1974) The electrocardiographic characteristics of the variant—Prinzmetal's—atypical form of angina pectoris manifesting in complicating ventricular extrasystoles. *S.A. Med. J.* **48,** 1146.

27 SCHERF D. (1935) Koronarerkrankungen. *Ergebn. inn. Kinderheick* **20,** 237.

28 SCHERF D. (1944) Alterations in the form of T waves with changes in heart rate. *Amer. Heart J.* **28,** 332.

29 SCHERF D. (1960) Development of the electrocardiographic exercise test. *Amer. J. Cardiol.* **5,** 433.

30 SCHERF D. & SCHAFFER A. I. (1952) The electrocardiographic exercise test. *Amer. Heart J.* **43,** 927.

31 SILVERMAN M. E. & FLAMM M. D. (1971) Variant angina pectoris. Anatomic findings and prognostic implications. *Ann. Intern. Med.* **75,** 339.

32 TULLOCH J. A. (1952) The electrocardiographic features of high postero-lateral myocardial infarction. *Brit. Heart J.* **14,** 379.

33 UNTERMAN J. B. & DE GRAFF A. C. (1948) Effect of exercise on the electrocardiogram (Master '2-step' test) in diagnosis of coronary insufficiency. *Amer. J. med. Sci.* **215,** 671.

34 WEYN A. S. & MARRIOTT H. J. L. (1962) the T-V1 taller than T-V6 pattern. Its potential value in the early recognition of myocardial disease. *Amer. Heart. J.* **10,** 764.

35 WHITING R. B., KLEIN M.D. & VAN DER VEER J. (1970) Variant angina pectoris. *New Engl. J. Med.* **282,** 709.

36 ZWILLINGER L. (1935) Die Digitaliseinwirkung auf das Arbeits-Elektrokardiogramm. *Med. Klin.* **30,** 977.

Chapter 3
Bundle Branch Block

Bundle branch block refers to a delay or block of conduction in the right or left main branches of the bundle of His.

RIGHT BUNDLE BRANCH BLOCK

In right bundle branch block the right ventricle is stimulated by the impulse from the left bundle branch which passes to the right side of the septum below the block and then to the right ventricle (Fig. 69, Vector 1). Activation of the right ventricle is thus delayed.

Depolarization of the septum thus occurs normally, viz. from left to right (Vector 1 of Fig. 69). This is followed by depolarization of the free wall of the left ventricle in the usual manner, viz. from right to left (Vector 2 of Fig. 69). Finally, the free wall of the right ventricle is depolarized by an impulse from left to right (Vector 3 of Fig. 69). This force is also directed anteriorly.

This final activation of the free wall of the right ventricle is *slow* and *anomalous* in character, tending to be longitudinal or tangential rather than transverse (endocardial–epicardial). It would seem that the Purkinje system is programmed for the rapid transmission of the activation process from a central distributing point which is normally subendocardial. Activation entering the system from another direction, i.e. within the myocardium, is also transmitted but in a bizarre, relatively slow and ineffective manner. As a result, the deflection resulting from this form of anomalous activation is relatively increased in magnitude and slow.

SUMMARY

Sequence of depolarization:
1. Left to right through the septum.
2. Right to left through the free wall of the left ventricle.
3. Left to right through the free wall of the right ventricle. This force is also directed anteriorly and is anomalous in character.

This sequence results in a widened and notched QRS complex—an

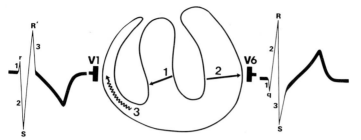

Fig. 69. Diagram illustrating ventricular depolarization in right bundle branch block, and its effect on a lead orientated to the right ventricle (lead V1) and a lead orientated to the left ventricle (lead V6).

rSR or M-shaped complex, in leads orientated to the right ventricle—usually leads V1 and V2 (Figs. 69, 70, 71, 72, 220 and 232). The proximal limb of the M-shaped complex—the R wave—is due to the stimulus spreading *towards* the electrode through the septum (Fig. 69, arrow 1). The S wave or notch in the M-shaped complex is due to the spread of the stimulus away from the electrode as it depolarizes the free wall of the left ventricle (Fig. 69, arrow 2). This force is always diminished in amplitude when compared with the S wave during normal intraventricular conduction. The R′ deflection—the distal limb of the M-shaped complex—is due to the anomalous spread of the stimulus through the free wall of the right ventricle towards the electrode (Fig. 69, arrow 3). As right ventricular depolarization occurs late, it is unopposed by left ventricular depolarization and therefore the right ventricular force will be fairly large. Further-

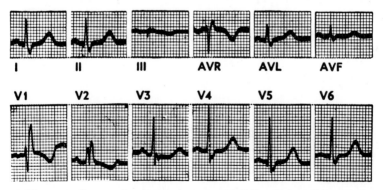

Fig. 70. Electrocardiogram showing the features of right bundle branch block. Note (*a*) the rSR′ M-shaped complex in the right ventricular leads—V1 and V2; and (*b*) the delayed and slurred S wave in the left ventricular leads—leads V4 to V6.

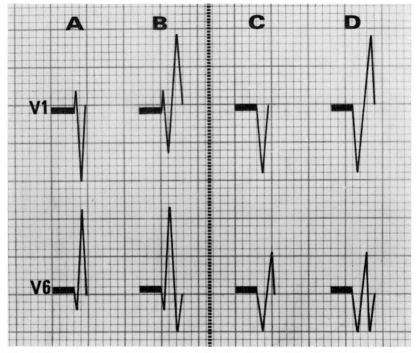

Fig. 71. Diagram illustrating the effect of right bundle branch block on the basic QRS pattern. Diagram A illustrates normal intraventricular conduction. Diagram B illustrates right bundle branch block. Diagram C illustrates myocardial infarction. Diagram D illustrates myocardial infarction complicated by right bundle branch (see text).

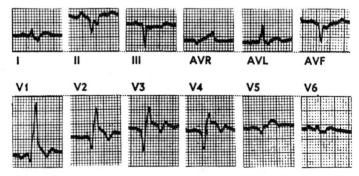

Fig. 72. Electrocardiogram illustrating the fully evolved phase of acute anteroseptal myocardial infarction complicated by right bundle branch block. Note (*a*) pathological Q waves in leads V2 to V5; (*b*) the terminal R' deflection in these leads; the R' deflection does not mask the pathological Q waves; (*c*) the raised coved S-T segments and low to inverted T waves in Standard lead I, lead AVL and leads V2 to V5.

more, depolarization of the free wall of the right ventricle does not necessarily proceed through the specialized conduction tissue, but through ordinary myocardial tissue (see above). This will result in a bizarre shape, and contribute to the height of, the R′ deflection.

Leads orientated to the left ventricle, usually leads V5 and V6, Standard lead I and AVL will show a **broad and slurred S wave** representing delayed anomalous right ventricle depolarization. This is due to the spread of the late right ventricular depolarization *away* from the electrode (Fig. 69, arrow 3; leads V4 to V6 in Fig. 70).

Because of the delayed and lengthened time of depolarization, the QRS complex is widened, viz. it is longer than 0.10 sec (greater than $2\frac{1}{2}$ small squares on the graph paper at the conventional paper speed of 25 mm per sec).

Empirically, right bundle branch block must satisfy at least two criteria: (1) there must be an R′ deflection in lead V1; and (2) there must be a delayed S wave in Standard lead I. This is an expression of a terminal QRS vector which is directed anteriorly and to the right.

The S-T segment and T wave are opposite in direction to the terminal QRS deflection. These are secondary phenomena, i.e. they occur secondary to the abnormal intraventricular conduction and do not indicate primary S-T segment or T wave abnormality). Thus, the rSR′ deflection in lead V1 will be associated with an inverted T wave; and the qRS deflection in lead V6 and Standard lead I will be associated with an upright T wave (Figs. 69 and 70).

Partial right bundle branch block is diagnosed when the QRS pattern is that of right bundle branch block but the QRS complexes are not widened beyond 0.10 sec.

Note: Right bundle branch block does not alter the *initial* deflection of the QRS complex. Thus, leads orientated to the right ventricle reflect the basic rS complex—the first part of the M-shaped complex (lead V1 in Diagram A of Fig. 71). Right bundle branch block merely results in the addition of an R′ deflection (lead V1 in Diagram B of Fig. 71). Leads orientated to the left ventricle reflect the normal initial qR complex (lead V6 in Diagram A of Fig. 71). Right bundle branch block merely results in the addition of a terminal slurred S wave (lead V6 in Diagram B of Fig. 71). The initial deflection of the QRS complex in right bundle branch block, therefore, reflects the form of intraventricular conduction before the advent of the right bundle branch block; abnormalities in the initial deflection of the QRS complex, e.g. those due to infarction or hypertrophy will, therefore, still be reflected in the presence of the complicating right bundle branch block. This principle is illustrated in Diagrams C and D of Fig.

71. Diagram C illustrates the pathological Q wave of myocardial infarction in leads V1 and V6. Diagram D illustrates the anterior infarction complicated by right bundle branch block.

Note: The initial part of the QRS complex is the same as in Diagram C, the only alterations are the addition of an R' deflection in lead V2 with a diminution of the S wave and a prominent slurred S wave in lead V6. A representative example of myocardial infarction complicated by right bundle branch block is illustrated in Fig. 72.

Note: These principles do *not* apply to left bundle branch block, for in this condition the initial QRS forces are markedly altered as a result of the block.

Significance of right bundle branch block

Right bundle branch block may occur in the following conditions:
1.   Occasionally, in normal individuals.
2.   As a transient phenomenon in acute pulmonary embolism (see Chapter 4).
3.   In coronary artery disease.
4.   Incomplete or complete right bundle branch block is found in 95 per cent of cases of atrial septal defect.
5.   As a manifestation of right ventricular diastolic overload (see Chapter 4).
6.   In active carditis, e.g. diphtheritic.

LEFT BUNDLE BRANCH BLOCK

In left bundle branch block the left ventricle is activated by the impulse from the right bundle branch which passes to the left side of the septum below the block (Vector 1a in Fig. 73). This activation process occurs near-synchronously with some activation of the free right ventricular wall in the right paraseptal region (Vector 1b of Fig. 73). This is followed by the activation process of the free wall of the right ventricle—a vector of small magnitude (Vector 2 of Fig. 73). This, in turn, is followed by the delayed anomalous activation of the free wall of the left ventricle (Vector 3 of Fig. 73).

Activation of the left side of the interventricular septum, the left septal mass, and the free wall of the left ventricle is *delayed* and *anomalous* in character. The anomalous activation process is an expression of slow, abnormal intramyocardial conduction. It has been shown that the Purkinje system is in fact used in this anomalous form of left bundle branch block activation, but the activation pro-

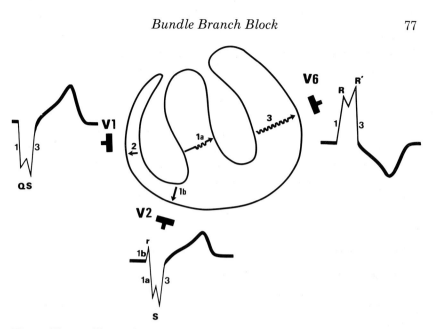

Fig. 73. Diagram illustrating ventricular depolarization in left bundle branch block, and its effect on a lead orientated to the right ventricle (lead V1), a lead orientated to the left ventricle (lead V6), and a lead orientated to the right paraseptal region (lead V2).

cess tends to be longitudinal, tangential or oblique, rather than centrifugal (an endocardial to epicardial spread). It would seem that the Purkinje system is programmed for the rapid transmission of the activation process from a central distributing point which is normally the left ventricular subendocardium. Activation entering the system from another direction, i.e. from *within* the myocardium, is also transmitted, but not in a very effective manner.

ELECTROCARDIOGRAPHIC MANIFESTATIONS

1.   *Prolonged QRS duration*

The QRS complex is prolonged to 0.12 sec or more, and may be as long as 0.20 sec. This is due to the delayed and anomalous activation of the left septal mass and the free wall of the left ventricle.

2.   *Effect on a lead orientated to the left ventricle*

Leads orientated to the left ventricle—usually leads V5, V6, AVL and Standard lead I—will reflect a wide, notched, *M- or plateau-shaped*

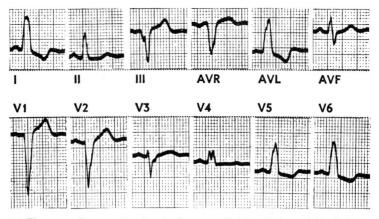

Fig. 74. Electrocardiogram showing the features of left bundle branch block. Note (*a*) the M-shaped or notched QRS complex in left ventricular leads—well seen in lead V4 but barely discernible in leads V5 and V6; and (*b*) the broad QS complex in the right ventricular leads—leads V1 and V2. The QRS duration is 0.12 sec (three small squares).

QRS complex: a wide notched R wave or an R-R' complex (Fig. 74). The proximal limb of the M-shaped complex results from the spread of the activation front towards the electrode, through the interventricular septum. The distal limb of the M-shaped complex is due to the spread of the activation front towards the electrode through the free wall of the left ventricle. There can be no initial q wave, no matter how small, in leads V5, V6 and Standard lead I in uncomplicated left bundle branch block.

3. *Effect on a lead orientated to the right ventricle*

The activation sequence will result in a wide and notched QS complex in a lead orientated to the right ventricle—lead V1 (Figs. 73 and 74). The proximal limb of the QRS complex is due to the spread of the activation front away from the electrode through the interventricular septum. The distal limb of the QRS complex is due to the spread of the activation front away from the electrode through the free wall of the left ventricle.

4. *Effect on a lead orientated to the right paraseptal region*

Leads orientated to the right paraseptal region—lead V2 and possibly lead V3—will reflect a small initial r wave followed by a deep, wide and notched S wave (Figs. 73 and 74). The initial r wave is due to the spread of the activation front through the right paraseptal region towards the electrode (Fig. 73). The deep, wide and notched S wave is due to the spread of the activation process away from the electrode through the interventricular septum and the free wall of the left ventricle.

5. *Secondary S-T segment and T wave changes*

The S-T segment and T wave are opposite in direction to the terminal QRS deflection. These are secondary phenomena, i.e. they occur secondarily to the abnormal intraventricular conduction and do not indicate primary S-T segment and T wave abnormality. Thus, in leads orientated to the left ventricle (leads V5 and V6) the S-T segment is depressed and often minimally convex-upward. The T wave is inverted with a blunt nadir (Figs. 73 and 74). The T wave is asymmetrical in leads orientated to the right ventricle (leads V1 and V2) the S-T segment is elevated and often minimally concave-upward. The T wave is upright, asymmetrical and with a relatively blunt apex (Figs. 73 and 74).

Significance of complete left bundle branch block

Complete left bundle branch block indicates *organic heart disease*. It is commonly associated with ischaemic and hypertensive heart disease.

ARBORIZATION BLOCK

Note: When bundle branch block (right or left) is associated with low amplitude complexes, the condition is sometimes referred to as **arborization block;** this form of bundle branch block has been incorrectly attributed to a block of the Purkinje fibres. The term is rarely used today.

Chapter 4
Ventricular Hypertrophy

LEFT VENTRICULAR HYPERTROPHY

The R wave of the qR complex recorded by a lead orientated to the left ventricle, and the S wave of the rS complex recorded by a lead orientated to the right ventricle, may indirectly be regarded as reflections of left ventricular depolarization (see Chapter 1; Fig. 8). In left ventricular hypertrophy these waves are exaggerated because of the increased electrical forces generated by the hypertrophied wall. Thus, **leads orientated to the left ventricle—usually leads V5 and V6, Standard lead I and lead AVL—will record tall R waves, and leads orientated to the right ventricle—V1 and V2—will record deep S waves** (Fig. 75).

If, in the adult, the sum of the S wave in lead V1 and the R wave in lead V6 exceeds 37 mm, the presence of left ventricular hypertrophy may usually be inferred, although these criteria may possibly be normal in a thin-chested individual.

In left ventricular hypertrophy depolarization of the left ventricular wall takes longer than normal. There is thus a **delay in the onset of the intrinsicoid deflection,** i.e. the time from the beginning of the QRS complex to the apex of the R wave (measured 'horizontally') is greater than 0.045 sec (Figs. 76, 77 and 241).

The normal initial q wave is frequently diminished in amplitude

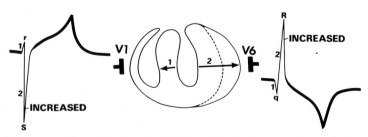

Fig. 75. Diagram illustrating the effect of left ventricular hypertrophy on a lead orientated to the right ventricle (lead V1), and a lead orientated to the left ventricle (lead V6).

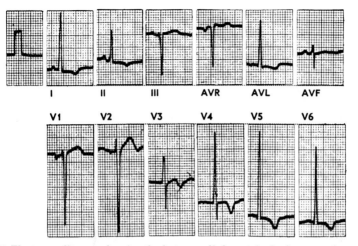

Fig. 76. Electrocardiogram showing the features of left ventricular hypertrophy and strain or left ventricular systolic overload. Note (*a*) the deep S waves in right ventricular leads—leads V1 and V2, and the tall R waves in left ventricular leads—leads V4 to V6; (*b*) the 'strain' pattern—depressed convex-upward S-T segment with inverted T wave—in left ventricular leads—leads V4 to V6; (*c*) the horizontal heart position—a qR complex in lead AVL; (*d*) the counter-clockwise rotation—rS complexes in leads V1 and V2, and qR complexes in leads V4 to V6; the transition zone is marked by the transition complex in lead V3; (*e*) the ventricular activation time as measured, for example, in lead AVL is 0.05 sec. (*f*) The QRS axis is directed at 0°; the T wave axis is directed at ± 180°.

and may disappear completely. This is probably an expression of associated incomplete left bundle branch block, and is only seen with left ventricular systolic overload (see page 90).

Leads orientated to the left ventricle may also reflect a **'strain' pattern**—a depressed convex-upwards S-T segment and an inverted T wave (Figs. 75 and 76; see also Fig. 55). This is an expression of left ventricular systolic overload (see page 90). The nadir of the T wave is relatively blunt and the limbs are asymmetrical. 'Strain' is a useful non-specific term signifying an abnormal state of the myocardium. It is possibly due to increased tension within the myocardium, or a result of the relative ischaemia resulting from the disproportion between the muscle mass and the available blood supply.

Left ventricular hypertrophy usually results in counter-clockwise rotation and, when of long-standing duration, is often associated with a horizontal heart or left axis deviation (Fig. 77). It must, however, be emphasized that left axis deviation is not synonymous with left ventricular hypertrophy. If, indeed, left axis deviation is associated with left ventricular hypertrophy, it reflects a complicat-

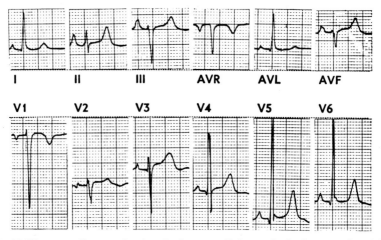

Fig. 77. Electrocardiogram showing the features of left ventricular hypertrophy with left ventricular diastolic overload. Note (*a*) the deep S wave in lead V1 and the tall R waves in leads V5 and V6; (*b*) the tall symmetrical T waves and slightly elevated concave-upward S-T segments in leads V5 and V6; (*c*) the well-marked q wave in leads V4 to V6 (compare with the q wave left ventricular systolic overload—Fig. 76); (*d*) the horizontal heart position—qR complex in lead AVL, and the counter-clockwise rotation—qR complexes in leads V4 to V6; the delay in the intrinsicoid deflection—ventricular activaton time, measured in left ventricular leads, is 0.05 sec.

ing intraventricular conduction defect. This is due to concomitant fibrosis—the result of long-standing hypertension—which interrupts the anterosuperior division of the left main bundle branch (see page 119). See Chapter 7 on the Electrical axis and also section on the Overload Concept (below). With left ventricular systolic overload (see page 90), the QRS axis is frequently directed at 0° and the T wave axis, in a diametrically opposite position, at ± 180°. See Chapter 7 and Fig. 121. Empirically, this means that lead AVF will reflect an equiphasic QRS complex and an equiphasic T wave, whereas Standard lead I will reflect a dominantly upright QRS complex and an inverted T wave (Fig. 76).

SUMMARY OF POSSIBLE ELECTROCARDIOGRAPHIC FINDINGS IN LEFT VENTRICULAR HYPERTROPHY

1. **Tall R waves** in leads V5 and V6, Standard lead I and lead AVL **Deep S waves** in leads V1 and V2.
2. **Delay in the onset of the intrinsicoid deflection.**
3. The **'Strain' pattern**—depressed, convex upward, S-T segment

with inverted asymmetrical T wave with blunt nadir in leads V5 and
V6, Standard lead I and lead AVL due to left ventricular systolic
overload (see also page 90).

4. **Counter-clockwise** rotation.
5. **Left axis deviation.**
    See also section on left ventricular diastolic overload (page 89).

RIGHT VENTRICULAR HYPERTROPHY

In right ventricular hypertrophy the dominant right ventricle
occupies the whole anterior surface of the heart resulting in
clockwise rotation. The electrocardiogram reflects a **vertical
position** or **right axis deviation** (Fig. 79).

Normally, depolarization of the interventricular septum occurs
first and is followed by depolarization of the free walls of both
ventricles (Figs. 6 and 7). The greater force of the left free wall
counteracts the weaker force of the right free wall (Fig. 8). In right
ventricular hypertrophy the potential force of the right ventricle—
particularly the crista supraventricularis—is greatly increased and
may even exceed that of the left free wall (Fig. 78). The R wave in right
ventricular leads (V1 to V4) may thus represent both septal and right
ventricular depolarization (Vectors 1a and 1b of Fig. 78) and,
consequently, is increased in amplitude. The tall R wave in lead V1,
in addition, usually reflects a small initial slur (Fig. 239).

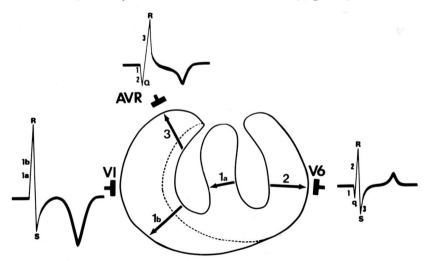

Fig. 78. Diagram illustrating the effect of right ventricular hypertrophy of leads V1,
V6 and AVR.

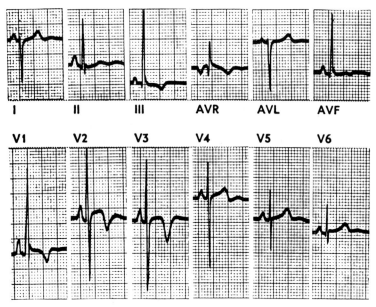

Fig. 79. Electrocardiogram showing the features of right ventricular hypertrophy and strain—right ventricular systolic overload; from a patient with the tetralogy of Fallot. Note (*a*) the tall R waves and 'strain' pattern in right ventricular leads—leads V1 to V4; (*b*) the vertical heart position—qR complex in lead AVF—and the clockwise rotation—RS or rS complexes in leads V1 to V5; (*c*) the tall peaked P waves—**P. congenitale**—in Standard lead II and lead VI; (*d*) The QRS axis is directed to + 130°; the T wave axis is directed to − 10°.

Leads facing the right ventricle may also record a **'strain'** pattern—a depressed convex-upward S-T segment with an inverted T wave (Figs. 78 and 79) (see also section on Right Ventricular Systolic Overload, page 91).

An S wave may be conspicuous in left ventricular leads due to late depolarization of a remote region of the right ventricle (Fig. 78). This force flows directly towards lead AVR—the right shoulder lead—and contributes towards a large R wave in that lead. It is also directed towards the negative poles of Standard leads I, II and III, and therefore inscribes an **S wave** in all three leads—this is termed the **S1, S2, S3 syndrome.** It probably reflects activation of the muscle in the right ventricular outflow tract—the **crista supraventricularis** (see also page 122).

The electrical activity of the crista supraventricularis adds greatly to the increased right ventricular forces and may even be the dominant contributing factor to the electrocardiographic manifestations of right ventricular hypertrophy.

SUMMARY OF POSSIBLE ELECTROCARDIOGRAPHIC FINDINGS IN RIGHT VENTRICULAR HYPERTROPHY

1. **Clockwise** rotation.
2. **Right axis deviation** or **vertical** heart position.
3. **Tall R waves** in **right ventricular leads.**
4. Small initial slur, notch or q wave in lead V1 (Fig. 239).
5. '**Strain**' pattern in **right ventricular leads.**
6. Tall R wave lead AVR.
7. The S1, S2, S3 syndrome.

See also section on the Overload Concept (below).

THE ELECTROCARDIOGRAPHIC MANIFESTATIONS OF RIGHT VENTRICULAR HYPERTROPHY IN VARIOUS CLINICAL CONDITIONS

Acute cor pulmonale

Acute cor pulmonale—due, for example, to acute and moderate to massive pulmonary embolism or, rarely, severe pneumonia—may manifest as follows:

Transient manifestations of the following:

1. The **S1, Q3, T3 pattern.** This is the classic presentation of moderate to large pulmonary embolism and manifests with a prominent S wave in Standard lead I, prominent Q wave and inverted T wave in Standard lead III (Fig. 80).
2. Inverted T waves over the right precordial leads—leads V1 to V3 or V4.
3. Coved and elevated S-T segments over the right precordial leads—leads V1 to V3 or V4 (Figs. 80 and 81). This is rare.
4. **Right axis deviation** (Fig. 80).
5. **Right ventricular hypertrophy and 'strain'** (as described above). This is uncommon.
6. **Right bundle branch block** (Fig. 81).
7. **P. pulmonale.**
8. **Sinus tachycardia.**

   Note: (*a*) The presentation of inverted T waves and possible

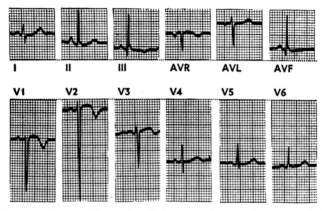

Fig. 80. Electrocardiogram illustrating the features of acute pulmonary embolism. Note (a) the S1, Q3, T3 pattern; (b) T wave inversion and slightly raised convex-upward S-T segments in leads V1 and V2; (c) the mean frontal plane QRS axis of + 90°.

elevated and coved S-T segments over the right precordial leads may resemble, or incorrectly suggest, a diagnosis of anteroseptal myocardial infarction. (b) The prominent Q wave and inverted T wave in Standard lead III may resemble, or incorrectly suggest, a diagnosis of inferior wall myocardial infarction. Thus, when on superficial examination, the electrocardiogram suggests the combination of inferior and anteroseptal infarctions (Fig. 81), the possibility of acute pulmonary embolism should be considered and must be excluded.

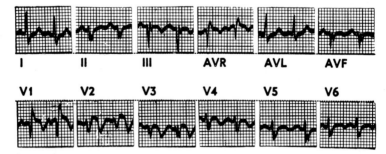

Fig. 81. Electrocardiogram showing the features of acute pulmonary embolism (autopsy revealed a pulmonary embolus in the left main pulmonary artery). Note (a) partial right bundle branch block—rR′ pattern in lead V1 and delayed S wave in leads V4 to V6; (b) the injury pattern—elevated coved S-T segments in leads V1 and V2, and to a lesser extent in leads AVF, V3, V4 and Standard lead III; (c) the inverted T waves in Standard lead III and leads AVF and V1 to V6; (d) sinus tachycardia.

DIFFERENTIAL DIAGNOSIS OF ACUTE PULMONARY EMBOLISM
AND MYOCARDIAL INFARCTION

Acute pulmonary embolism

The changes are transient, often lasting a few hours only.
Q wave in Standard lead II, insignificant, absent or rare.
An injury pattern of coved, elevated S-T segments may appear in
leads V1 to V3 but is uncommon or rare in leads V4, V5 and V6.
Always associated with sinus tachycardia.

Inferior myocardial infarction

Changes usually last for many days or weeks.
A prominent or pathological Q wave is always present in Standard
lead II and lead AVF.

Anteroseptal myocardial infarction

The injury pattern of elevated and coved S-T segment usually extends
beyond lead V3, i.e. usually from leads V1 to V5.

Infarction may be associated with sinus tachycardia or sinus
bradycardia or a normal sinus rhythm.

Chronic cor pulmonale—emphysema

The electrocardiographic manifestations of chronic cor pulmonale—
emphysema (Fig. 83) are due to:
1. Right ventricular dominance.
2. The downward displacement of the heart secondary to downward
displacement of the diaphragm (Fig. 82).
3. The lowered electrical transmission resulting from the surrounding voluminous lung.

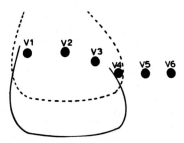

Fig. 82. Diagram illustrating the effect of the
downward displacement of the heart in
emphysema on the electrode relationship.
The precordial electrodes become orientated
to the upper or basal regions of the heart.

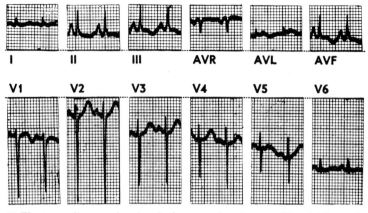

Fig. 83. Electrocardiogram showing the features of emphysema. Note (*a*) the tendency to low voltage in the extremity leads and leads V5 and V6; (*b*) the clockwise rotation—rS complexes in leads V1 to V5; (*c*) the tall peaked P waves—**P. pulmonale**—in lead AVF and Standard leads II and III; absence of the tall R waves in the right precordial leads which are usually associated with right ventricular hypertrophy.

This may result in:

1.   P pulmonale—tall peaked P waves in Standard leads II and III and lead AVF. The frontal plane P wave axis is usually directed at $+90°$ (see page 102).

2.   A sloping P-R segment: the effect of the increased Tp deflection (see page 48).

3.   Vertical heart position or right axis deviation and clockwise rotation expressions of right ventricle hypertrophy.

4.   Low voltage; particularly in the extremity leads and leads V5 and V6: the effect of the lowered electrical transmission resulting from the surrounding emphysematous lung (Fig. 83). Other causes of low voltage are considered on page 298.

5.   A tendency to rS patterns throughout the precordial leads (Fig. 83). This is due to the downward displacement of the heart and diaphragm (Fig. 82). As a result, the precordial leads are orientated to the upper or basal regions of the heart which usually reflects rS patterns.

The 'Standard lead I sign' of emphysema

Inspection of Standard lead I alone frequently suggests the diagnosis of emphysema, since all deflections or impressions are *minimal* and

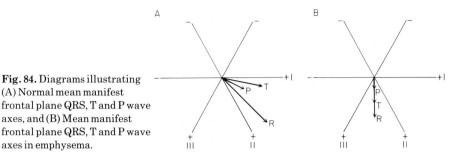

Fig. 84. Diagrams illustrating (A) Normal mean manifest frontal plane QRS, T and P wave axes, and (B) Mean manifest frontal plane QRS, T and P wave axes in emphysema.

equiphasic on this lead (Fig. 83). This manifestation is due to the following (Fig. 84):

1. The frontal plane P wave axis is emphysema is usually directed at +90° resulting in a minimal or equiphasic deflection in Standard lead I (see Chapter 7).

2. The frontal plane QRS axis is usually directed at +90° resulting in a minimum or equiphasic deflection in Standard lead I.

3. The frontal plane T wave axis is directed either at +90° or −90° resulting in a minimal or equiphasic deflection in Standard lead I.

4. The voltage is diminished.

THE OVERLOAD CONCEPT

In the early 1950s, a concept arose attempting to correlate the various patterns of ventricular hypertrophy with cardiac haemodynamics. Cabrera & Monroy (1952)[1] indicated that ventricular hypertrophy could occur as a result of strain or overload either in systole or diastole, and this could result in different electrocardiographic manifestations. This is known as the 'overload concept'. It should be noted, however, that absolute haemodynamic-electrocardiographic correlation is by no means invariable. Indeed, the validity of the concept has been challenged. Nevertheless, the concept cannot be dismissed entirely and, at very least, forms a useful guide.

DIASTOLIC OVERLOAD

Diastolic overload occurs when there is an **increased flow into either ventricle.** *The overfilling of the ventricle* causes an increased stretch and strain (or overload) of the myocardial fibre in diastole.

Left ventricular diastolic overload occurs in:

mitral incompetence
aortic incompetence
ventricular septal defect $\left\{\begin{array}{l}\text{the left to right shunt results in an}\\\text{increased return to the left ventricle.}\end{array}\right.$
patent ductus arteriosus

Right ventricular diastolic overload occurs in:

atrial septal defect $\left\{\begin{array}{l}\text{the left to right shunt results in an}\\\text{increased flow to the right ventricle.}\end{array}\right.$

tricuspid incompetence

SYSTOLIC OVERLOAD

Systolic overload occurs when there is an **abnormal resistance to outflow** from either ventricle.

Left ventricular systolic overload occurs in:

systemic hypertension
aortic stenosis
coarctation of the aorta

Right ventricular systolic overload occurs in:

pulmonary hypertension
pulmonary embolism
pulmonary stenosis

ELECTROCARDIOGRAPHIC FEATURES

The diagnosis of **left** ventricular systolic and diastolic overload is made from *leads orientated to the* **left** *ventricle*, viz. leads V5 and V6, Standard lead I and lead AVL, while that of **right** ventricular systolic and diastolic overload is made from *leads orientated to the* **right** *ventricle*, viz. leads V1 and V2 (Fig. 85).

Left ventricular overload patterns

Left ventricular systolic overload (Figs. 76 and 85)

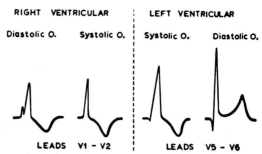

Fig. 85. Diagram illustrating the patterns of left and right ventricular systolic and diastolic overload.

This is characterized by:
1. Tall R waves (usually not as tall as found in left ventricular diastolic overload)
2. Delay in the onset of the intrinsicoid deflection (longer than 0.045 sec)
3. The left ventricular 'strain' pattern
    (a) Depressed convex-upward S-T segment
    (b) Inverted T waves
4. Diminution in amplitude or disappearance of the normal small initial q wave. This is probably due to associated incomplete left bundle branch block.

in leads V5 and V6, Standard lead I and lead AVL.

Left ventricular diastolic overload (Figs. 77 and 85)

This is characterized by:
1. Tall R waves
2. Prominent, deep but narrow initial q or Q waves[2]
3. Tall peaked T waves
4. Slight concave-upward elevation of the S-T segment

in leads V5 and V6, Standard lead I and lead AVL

Right ventricular overload patterns

Right ventricular diastolic overload

This is characterized by classical right bundle branch block (Fig. 70).

Right ventricular systolic overload (Fig. 79)

This is characterized by:
1. Tall R waves
2. Delay in the intrinsicoid deflection
3. Right ventricular 'strain' pattern
    (*a*) depressed convex-upward S-T
        segments
    (*b*) inverted T waves.

    in leads V1 and V2.

REFERENCES

1 CABRERA C. E. & MONROY J. R. (1952) Systolic and diastolic loading of the heart. *Amer. Heart J.* **43,** 661.
2 WATSON D. G. & KEITH J. D. (1962) The Q wave in lead V6 in heart disease of infancy and childhood, with special reference to diastolic loading. *Amer. Heart J.* **63,** 629.

Chapter 5
Drug and Electrolyte Effect

DIGITALIS EFFECT

Digitalis **shortens the Q-T interval** and consequently alters the S-T segment in a characteristic manner. The **S-T segment is depressed** with a straight, gradual, downward slope ending in a terminal rise to the isoelectric level; it may be likened to the **mirror-image of a correction or check mark** (Figs. 43, 86 and 87).

This effect is usually seen in leads with the tallest R wave, usually Standard leads I and II, and leads V4 to V6. This manifestation suggests digitalis administration and does not necessarily indicate digitalis intoxication. When the characteristic S-T segment change appears in nearly all leads, i.e. in leads without tall R waves (leads recording rS complexes) as well as leads with tall R waves, the tracing is suggestive of digitalis toxicity. This is usually a late and uncommon sign of digitalis toxicity.

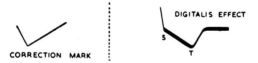

Fig. 86. Diagram illustrating digitalis effect on the S-T segment, viz. a gradual downward slope with a sharp terminal rise—the mirror-image of a correction mark.

EFFECT OF DIGITALIS ON BASIC NORMAL AND BASIC ABNORMAL S-T SEGMENTS AND T WAVES

If the S-T segment and T wave are normal or relatively normal *before* the administration of digitalis, the sharp terminal rise of the distal limb of the T wave will rise *above* the baseline following the administration of digitalis (A of Fig. 87). In the case of pre-existing abnormal S-T segments or T waves, however (i.e. low to inverted T waves associated with depressed S-T segments), the distal limb of the T wave will *not* rise above the baseline (B of Fig. 87). See also the effects of digitalis on the QRS-T angle (page 126).

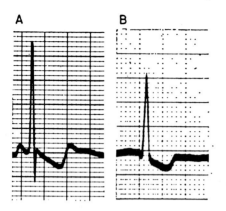

Fig. 87. (A) Lead V5. QRST complex illustrating digitalis *effect.* Note the gradual downward slope of the S-T segment and the sharp upward terminal deflection of the T wave which rises above the baseline. This indicates that the T wave was probably normal before the administration of digitalis. (B) Lead V5. QRST complex illustrating digitalis effect superimposed on pre-existing T wave abnormality. Note the terminal limb of the T wave does *not* rise above the baseline. This indicates that the T wave was probably abnormal before the administration of digitalis.

THE DISORDERS OF CARDIAC RHYTHM ASSOCIATED WITH DIGITALIS ADMINISTRATION

Digitalis administration may be associated with any arrhythmia except the Type II (Mobitz Type II) second degree A-V block. Some typical examples are listed below and described in detail in Chapters 10 to 17.

The commonest manifestations of digitalis toxicity are (1) **bi-geminal rhythm due to alternate ventricular extrasystoles,** and (2) **paroxysmal atrial tachycardia with irregular Type I second degree A-V block.**

<table>
<tr><td align="center">*Digitalis effect*</td><td align="center">*Digitalis toxicity*</td></tr>
<tr><td>sinus bradycardia</td><td>ventricular extrasystoles</td></tr>
<tr><td>1st degree A-V block complicating normal sinus rhythm</td><td>atrial extrasystoles</td></tr>
<tr><td>2nd degree A-V block complicating normal sinus rhythm</td><td>paroxysmal atrial tachycardia with varying Type I 2nd degree A-V block</td></tr>
<tr><td></td><td>multifocal ventricular extrasystoles</td></tr>
<tr><td></td><td>paroxysmal ventricular tachycardia</td></tr>
</table>

Factors which predispose to digitalis toxicity

1.   *Diseased heart*: the more advanced the heart disease, the less the tolerance to digitalis.
2.   *Hypopotassaemia*: Hypopotassaemia will predispose to digitalis toxicity. This usually results from the concomitant administration of thiazide diuretics.
3.   *Diminished metabolism of digitalis*: this is particularly prone to occur in cases of *renal* and *hepatic* disease.

POTASSIUM EFFECT

HYPERKALAEMIA

The following electrocardiographic sequence is associated with a progressive rise in the serum potassium level (Figs. 88 and 89).

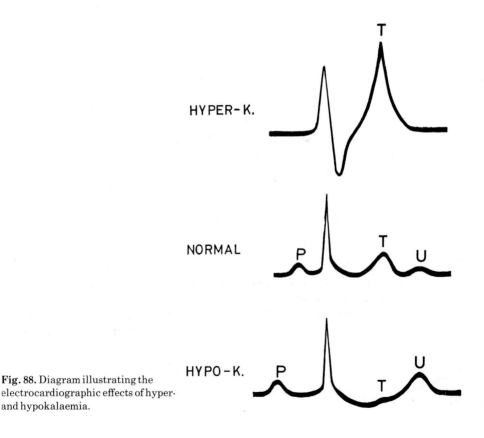

Fig. 88. Diagram illustrating the electrocardiographic effects of hyper- and hypokalaemia.

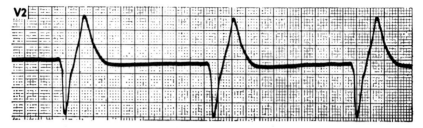

Fig. 89. The electrocardiogram (lead V2) shows: 1. A slow ventricular rhythm: rate = 28 beats per minute. 2. The features of hyperkalaemia: (*a*) absent P waves, (*b*) bizarre, low-amplitude, QRS complexes, (*c*) tall, wide, symmetrical T wave, (*d*) 'blending' of the QRS and T deflections to form large, bizarre, biphasic complexes.

1. The T wave becomes tall and peaked.
2. There is diminution in the amplitude of the R wave.
3. The QRS complex becomes widened.
4. The QRS complex blends with the T wave producing a wide, bizarre, diphasic deflection, so that it becomes difficult to detect an S-T segment.
5. There is progressive diminution in the amplitude of the P wave which eventually disappears.

HYPOKALAEMIA

With a progressive diminution in the serum potassium level the following sequence of abnormal electrocardiography occurs (Figs. 88, 90, 91 and 92):

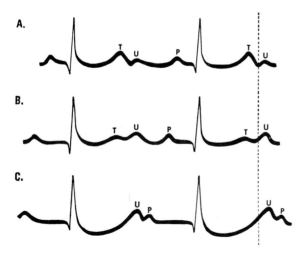

Fig. 90. Diagrams illustrating the electrocardiographic manifestations of progressive hypokalaemia. *Note*: increasing prominence of the U wave; diminishing amplitude of the T wave; increasing P-R interval; constancy of the Q–T interval (dotted line).

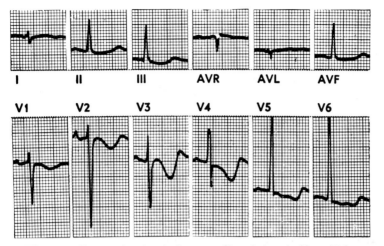

Fig. 91. Electrocardiogram showing the features of hypokalaemia. Note: (*a*) depressed S-T segments in most leads; (*b*) prominent U waves in Standard leads II and III, and leads AVF and V2 to V6; the U wave, at first glance, appears to be the T wave; the T wave, however, is seen in leads V5 and V6 as a small, rounded positive deflection on the terminal part of the S-T segment; the prominent U wave, if mistaken for a T wave, gives the false impression of a prolonged Q–T interval.

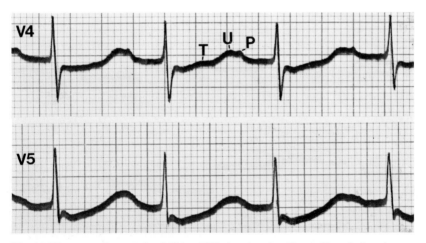

Fig. 92. Electrocardiogram (leads V4 and V5) showing the effects of hypokalaemia. Note (*a*) the prominent U wave; (*b*) the virtual disappearance of the T wave which is barely discernible in lead V4 and completely absent in lead V5; (*c*) the prolonged P-R interval of 0.26 sec; (*d*) the depressed S-T segment. Note, too, how the prominent U wave could be mistaken for a T wave and, thereby, leading to an erroneous conclusion of the presence of a prolonged Q-T interval.

1. The **U wave becomes prominent.**
2. The **T wave becomes flattened and finally inverted.** The very prominent associated U wave may thus be mistaken for a T wave, and the Q–U interval may be mistaken for a prolonged Q–T interval.
3. The **S-T segment becomes depressed.**
4. The **P-R interval becomes prolonged.** When this occurs, the P wave shifts closer to the prominent U wave and may eventually be superimposed on the U wave (Figs. 90 and 92). Under this circumstance, the P wave may be mistaken for a normal U wave and thereby further favouring the possible misinterpretation of the prominent U wave as a T wave.
5. Very rarely, there may be a complicating S-A block.

CALCIUM EFFECT

HYPOCALCAEMIA

Hypocalcaemia manifests with a **prolonged Q-T interval** (Figs. 93 and 94). This is due solely to a prolongation of the S-T segment which becomes horizontal and isoelectric, 'hugging' the baseline for a relatively long period. This horizontality may mimic the horizontality of the S-T segment which is associated with coronary insufficiency (see page 45).

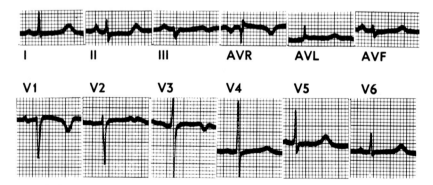

Fig. 93. The electrocardiogram was recorded from a woman with hypoparathyroidism and a low serum calcium. It shows the following features: (*a*) There is a prolonged Q–T interval. The Q–Tc was calculated to be 56.5 sec. (*b*) The prolongation of the Q–T interval is due to a prolongation of the S-T segment. Note that the T wave is not particularly widened. Note, too, that the S-T segment reflects marked horizontality and is isoelectric, hugging the baseline for 6 mm, a relatively long period of 0.24 sec. There is also a tendency to a sharp-angled ST-T junction.

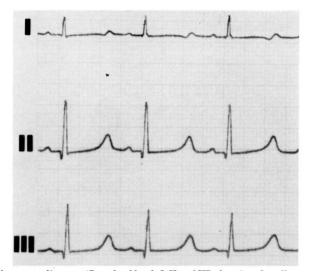

Fig. 94. Electrocardiogram (Standard leads I, II and III) showing the effects of hypocalcaemia. Note the prolonged Q-T interval due to prolongation of the S-T segment. The Q-Tc = 0.58 sec.

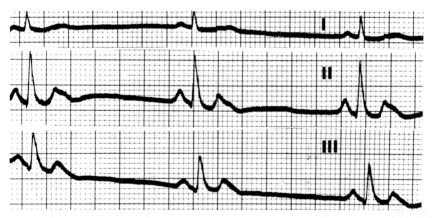

Fig. 95. Electrocardiogram (Standard leads I, II and III) was recorded from a patient with a parathyroid adenoma and reflects the features of hypercalcaemia. There is sinus rhythm complicated by alternate blocked atrial extrasystoles. The P′ waves of the atrial extrasystoles are superimposed upon and distort the S-T segments. None of these P′ waves is associated with an ensuing QRS complex. The coupling interval of P′ wave to the preceding P wave is very short and measures 0.31 sec. The Q-T interval is very short and measures 0.40 sec. The Q-Tc is also very short and measures 0.34 sec. Note that blocked alternate atrial extrasystoles result in a slow regular ventricular rhythm.

HYPERCALCAEMIA

Hypercalcaemia manifests with a **shortened Q-T interval** (Fig. 95).

QUINIDINE EFFECT

Quinidine has the following electrocardiographic effects:

1. **The QRS complex is widened.** If the increase in the width of the QRS complex is greater than 25 per cent of the QRS complex in the tracing recorded before quinidine administration, it reflects a toxic effect and the quinidine must be stopped.
2. **The Q-T interval is lengthened.**
3. **The T wave becomes widened, notched, and low to inverted.**

Chapter 6
The P Wave: Atrial Activation

The P wave reflects atrial depolarization and is recorded as soon as the impulse leaves the S-A node.

Because the S-A node is situated in the right atrium, right atrial activation begins first and is followed shortly thereafter by left atrial activation (Fig. 98). The two processes overlap, as left atrial activation begins before the end of right atrial activation.

The electrocardiographic effects of atrial activity are best seen in Standard lead II and lead V1 or lead MCL1 (Fig. 230). When there is left axis deviation of the P wave, the abnormal P wave changes are best observed in Standard lead I.

ATRIAL ACTIVITY AS REFLECTED IN STANDARD LEAD II

When viewed in the frontal plane both the initial and terminal atrial forces are directed roughly parallel to the Standard lead II axis (see Chapter 7 for direction of the Standard lead II axis). Both forces thus record roughly the same deflection in this lead. And since both activation processes overlap (Fig. 96), a P wave is produced that

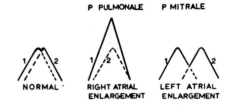

Fig. 96. Diagram illustrating the normal and abnormal components of the P wave as reflected in Standard lead II. (1) Right atrial component; (2) left atrial component.

theoretically has a small notched apex. Due to the close overlap of the two forces, however, this notch is rarely seen and the P wave is consequently pyramid-shaped with a smooth relatively blunt apex (A in Fig. 96). The amplitude in Standard lead II should not exceed 2.5 mm.

101

RIGHT ATRIAL ENLARGEMENT

With right atrial enlargement, the first, or right atrial component of the P wave is accentuated, resulting in a **tall P wave** with a **sharply pointed** or **peaked vertex** (Figs. 96, 97C and 101B). This P wave is often referred to as **P. pulmonale** or **P. congenitale** for it is frequently associated with the right atrial strain that is found in pulmonary hypertension and cyanotic congenital heart disease (see also pages 136 and 291).

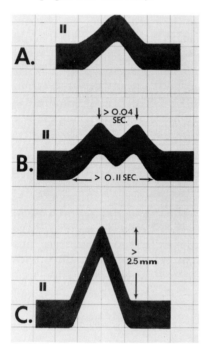

Fig. 97. Diagrammatic illustration of: (A) a normal P wave in Standard lead II, (B) the P wave of left atrial enlargement and (C) the P wave of right atrial enlargement.

LEFT ATRIAL ENLARGEMENT

With left atrial enlargement, the second, or terminal component of the P wave, representing left atrial activation, is *delayed* resulting in a **wide and notched P wave** exceeding 0.11 sec in duration (Fig. 96, B of Fig. 97 and A of Fig. 100). The duration of the notch, i.e. the interval between the 'camel humps' exceeds 0.04 sec. This P wave is often referred to as **P. mitrale** because of its frequent association with mitral valvular disease. Since there is frequent left axis deviation of the P wave (see page 137), this manifestation is frequently best seen in Standard lead I or lead AVL.

ATRIAL ACTIVITY AS REFLECTED IN LEAD V1

The right atrium is situated anteriorly in the thorax and to the right
of the ventricles (Fig. 98). The left atrium is situated more posteriorly
in the thorax, behind the ventricles (Fig. 98).

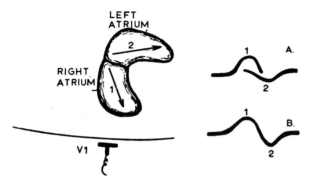

Fig. 98. Diagram illustrating the normal components of the P wave as reflected in lead
V1.

The right atrial force is directed towards lead V1 and thus the first
or right atrial component of the P wave is upright in lead V1 (Fig.
98A). The left atrial force is directed a little away from lead V1, and
thus the second, or left atrial component is only slightly negative in
this lead (Fig. 98A). As the two atrial forces overlap, the result is a P
wave that is mainly upright with a slight terminal negative or
equiphasic deflection (Fig. 98B). The normal P wave in lead V1 is thus
diphasic with but a shallow, terminal negative component.

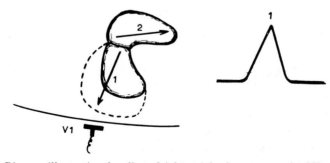

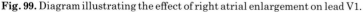

Fig. 99. Diagram illustrating the effect of right atrial enlargement on lead V1.

RIGHT ATRIAL ENLARGEMENT

With right atrial enlargement, the right atrial component is increased, resulting in a **tall peaked P wave** (Figs. 99, 101B) (see also page 136).

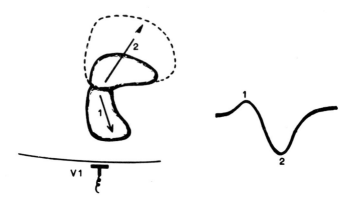

Fig. 100. Diagram illustrating the effect of left atrial enlargement on lead V1.

LEFT ATRIAL ENLARGEMENT

With left atrial enlargement, the magnitude of the left atrial component of the P wave is increased, delayed, and directed away from lead V1 (Fig. 100). The result is a P wave with a markedly **negative** and delayed terminal component (Figs. 100 and 101A).

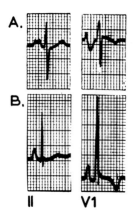

Fig. 101. Electrocardiograms showing the features of left and right atrial enlargement. (A) Left atrial enlargement (B) right atrial enlargement.

SUMMARY

P wave in:

	Standard lead II and/or Standard lead I	*Lead V1*
Right atrial enlargement	Tall and peaked	Tall and peaked
Left atrial enlargement	Wide and notched	Diphasic with negative terminal component

RETROGRADE ATRIAL ACTIVATION

Retrograde activation of the atria can occur with impulses of A-V nodal and ventricular origin (see Chapters 14 and 15). Retrograde activation may also occur in certain forms of reciprocal rhythm where the sinus impulse enters an A-V nodal by-pass and returns retrograde to activate the atria a second time.

With retrograde activation of the atria, the activation front is directed cranially, i.e. away from the positive poles of Standard leads II and III, and lead AVF. These leads will consequently reflect negative P′ deflections (Figs. 152, 160 and 226). The P′ wave in lead V1 is usually narrow, sharply pointed and positive and thus differs from the normal diphasic sinus P wave reflected by this lead (Figs. 102B and 228). See also section on P wave axis in Chapter 7, page 137.

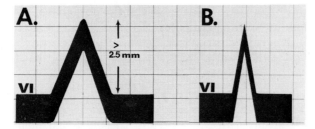

Fig. 102. Diagrammatic illustration of: (A) the P wave of right atrial enlargement in lead VI, and (B) the P′ wave in lead V1 of retrograde atrial activation due to an impulse arising within, or passing through, the A-V node.

Chapter 7
The Electrical Axis

Electrocardiographic diagnosis may be both empirical and deductive. Empirical diagnosis is based on clinical-electrocardiographic, as well as pathological-electrocardiographic correlation. For example, an inverted T wave in a particular lead, or a tall R wave in a particular lead, becomes known to be associated with a certain clinical or pathological state, and thereby assumes a diagnostic significance. Deductive electrocardiographic diagnosis is based on the orientation of electrocardiographic forces or vectors; e.g. the P wave, QRS complex, S-T segment, T wave and U wave vectors. This deductive vectorial method, in its simplest form, involves an analysis of the mean frontal plane P, QRS, T wave and U wave axes. It must be stressed that the empirical and deductive methods complement each other and both are, and should be, used in clinical electrocardiology. This chapter serves as an introduction to the determination and evaluation of frontal plane axes.

THE LEAD AXIS

Every electrocardiographic lead has a negative and a positive pole, and the location of these poles is termed the **polarity of the lead.** A hypothetical line joining the poles of a lead is known as the **axis of the lead.** Every lead axis is orientated in a certain direction depending upon the location of the positive and negative electrodes.

THE ELECTRICAL FIELD OF THE HEART

The heart is situated in the centre of the electrical field which it generates. The intensity of this electrical field diminishes algebraically with the distance from its centre. Thus the electrical intensity recorded by an electrode diminishes rapidly when the electrode is moved a short distance from the heart, and less and less as the electrode is moved still further away from the heart. With distances greater than 15 cm from the heart, the decrement in the intensity of the electrical field is hardly noticeable. Consequently, all electrodes placed at a distance greater than 15 cm from the heart may, in an electrical sense, be considered to be *equidistant* from the heart. For example, an electrode placed at 25 cm from the heart will record about the same potential as one placed 35 cm from the heart.

THE ORIENTATION OF THE LEAD AXES

THE STANDARD LEADS

Using this principle, Einthoven* deliberately placed the electrodes of the three Standard leads as far away from the heart as possible, i.e. on the extremities—the right arm, left arm and left leg. *These three electrodes are thus electrically equidistant from the heart.*

The leads derived from these three electrodes are conventionally as follows:

Standard lead I   Derived from electrodes on the right arm (negative pole) and left arm (positive pole) (Figs. 103 and 106).

Standard lead II   Derived from electrodes on the right arm (negative pole) and left leg (positive pole) (Figs. 104 and 106).

Standard lead III Derived from electrodes on the left arm (negative pole) and the left leg (positive pole) (Figs. 105 and 106).

The lead axes of these three leads form a triangle (Fig. 106A) and as the electrodes of these leads are regarded as equidistant from the heart, *the lead axes too may be considered to be equidistant from the*

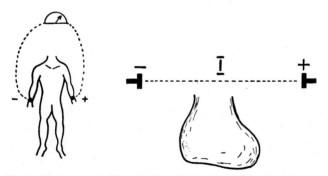

Fig. 103. Electrode placement of Standard lead I. Positive pole on the left arm.

* Willem Einthoven, physiologist of Leyden (1860–1927); inventor of the string galvanometer.

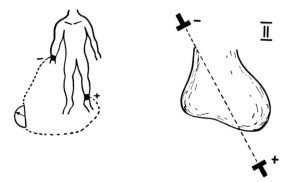

Fig. 104. Electrode placement of Standard lead II. Positive pole on the left leg.

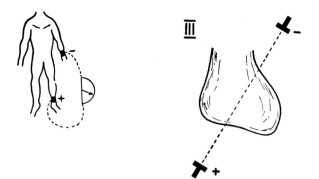

Fig. 105. Electrode placement of Standard lead III. Positive pole on the left leg.

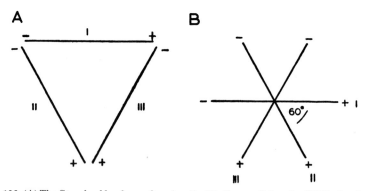

Fig. 106. (A) The Standard lead axes forming the Einthoven Triangle. (B) The lead axes of the Einthoven Triangle redrawn to form a triaxial reference system. *Note*: the orientation and polarity of each lead axis remain the same.

heart. These lead axes thus form an *equilateral triangle* with the heart at the centre (Fig. 106A)—the **Einthoven Triangle.**

To facilitate the graphic representation of the cardiac impulses, the three lead axes of the Einthoven Triangle may be redrawn so that they pass through the same zero or mid-point (Fig. 106B). The three lead axes thus bisect each other forming a triaxial system with each of the lead axes separated by 60° from one another.

Note: The polarity and orientation of the lead axes remains the same.

THE UNIPOLAR LIMB HEADS

A unipolar limb lead is derived as follows: the positive pole of the lead is attached to one of the limbs, and the negative pole is attached by three wires to all three limb electrodes. The *sum* of the three limb leads is at all times equal to *zero* potential. Thus, if these three leads are connected to a central terminal the potential of the terminal will be zero (see Appendix, page 310 and Figs. 254 and 255). A unipolar limb lead thus consists of a positive pole on one of the limbs and a negative pole at zero potential. Zero potential is located in the centre of the Einthoven Triangle since the centre of an equilateral triangle is equidistant from all its apices (Fig. 106A). The axis of a unipolar limb lead is, therefore, the hypothetical line drawn from the limb—right shoulder, left shoulder or left hip—to the centre of the Einthoven Triangle (Fig. 107A).

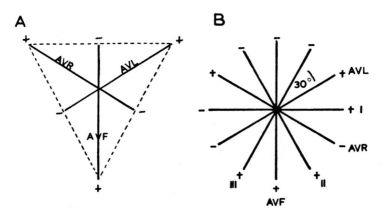

Fig. 107. (A) The triaxial reference system formed by the unipolar extremity leads. (B) The combination of the triaxial reference systems of the Standard and unipolar leads to form a hexaxial reference system.

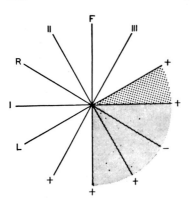

Fig. 108. The hexaxial reference system. Dark shading (0° to +90°) represents the normal range for frontal plane QRS axes. Light shading (0° to −29°) represents the range for slight left axis deviation.

These three unipolar lead axes also form a triaxial reference system with the axes 60° apart.

When the triaxial system of the Standard leads and the triaxial system of the unipolar limb leads are combined, they form a **hexaxial reference system** (Figs. 107A, 108 and 109). The triaxial system formed by the unipolar limb leads bisects the angles of the triaxial system formed by the Standard leads and the resulting hexaxial reference system divides the frontal plane into 30° intervals. By an irrational convention (see below), all degrees in the upper hemisphere of the hexaxial reference system are labelled negative degrees, and all degrees in the lower hemisphere are labelled positive degrees (Figs. 107B and 109). Thus, commencing at the positive end of the Standard lead I axis (labelled 0°) and progressing counter-clockwise, the leads will be successively at −30°, −60°, −90°, −120°, −150°, −180°. Progressing clockwise, from the positive pole of Standard lead I, the leads will be successively at +30°, +60°, +90°, +120°, +150°, +180°.

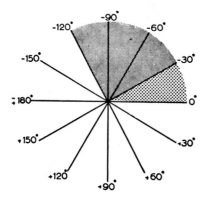

Fig. 109. The hexaxial reference system. Light shading (0° to −29°) represents the range of slight left axis deviation. Dark shading (−29° to −120°) represents the range of significant left axis deviation.

Note. The irrational convention of labelling the hexaxial reference system as positive and negative units must not be confused with the positive and negative poles of the lead axes.

It will also be noted that, with one exception, the positive poles of the lead axes are located from −30° clockwise to +120°. The exception is the negative pole of lead AVR which is located at +30° (Figs. 107B and 108).

THE MEAN ELECTRICAL AXIS

Excitation or depolarization spreads from one region of the heart to the other in the form of an advancing wave front. This may be represented by a number of forces (Fig. 110). In Chapter 1 the electrical activity of the ventricles was, for purposes of exposition, represented in a simplified form by two forces, viz. a small initial force from left to right, followed by a larger force from right to left (Fig. 8). In reality, however, the activation process consists of a number of

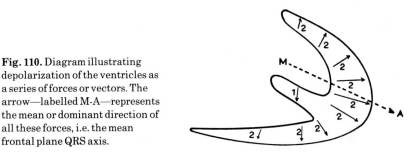

Fig. 110. Diagram illustrating depolarization of the ventricles as a series of forces or vectors. The arrow—labelled M-A—represents the mean or dominant direction of all these forces, i.e. the mean frontal plane QRS axis.

consecutive forces as shown in Fig. 110. The *general, average* or *dominant direction* of these forces is known as the *mean manifest frontal plane electrical axis* and is represented in Fig. 110 by the single force labelled M-A. This is, in effect, the electrical centre of gravity.

GRAPHING THE ELECTRICAL AXIS

If an impulse runs parallel to the axis of a lead, the force it generates will record the maximum deflection in the lead. The situation may be likened to an imaginary shadow—representing the amount of deflection—cast by the force on the lead axis (Fig. 111). If the direction of the force is towards the positive pole of the lead (A in Fig. 111 (X)) the deflection will be maximal and positive; if the force is towards the negative pole of the lead (B in Fig. 111 (X)) the deflection will be maximal and negative. Thus, in either case, the deflection will

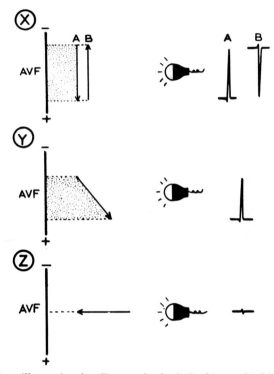

Fig. 111. Diagram illustrating the effect on a lead axis (in this case lead AVF) of forces or vectors orientated in various directions. A light source is directed at the lead axis and the imaginary 'shadow' cast by the vector on the lead axis represents the size of the deflection that will be recorded by that lead.

be maximal when compared with those recorded in other lead axes.

Such an impulse, electrical force or activation front that has both magnitude and direction is known as a *vector*.

If an impulse runs obliquely to the axis of a lead the deflection—or the shadow cast—on that lead will be less than that caused when the impulse travels parallel to the lead (Fig. 111 (Y)). The more oblique the approach to the lead, the less will be the deflection on that lead.

If the impulse runs at right angles to the axis of a lead, the deflection, or 'shadow' cast, on that lead will be nil—it is usually a small equiphasic deflection (Fig. 111 (Z)).

Note. The *net* positive or *net* negative deflection in any lead is gained by subtracting the smaller deflection above or below the baseline from the larger deflection above or below the baseline, e.g. the net positive deflection in A of Fig. 111 (X) will be the tall R wave minus the small q wave.

DETERMINATION OF THE MEAN ELECTRICAL AXIS

To determine the mean frontal plane QRS electrical axis the following procedure may be adopted:

(a) With reference to Fig. 112

Examine the *six frontal plane leads* I, II, III, AVR, AVL and AVF. Find the lead with the *smallest* and most *equiphasic* deflection. This is lead AVL in Fig. 112. On principles enunciated above, the electrical axis must run at *right angles to lead A VL*, and it must run *parallel to Standard lead II* (refer to Fig. 111). The deflection must, therefore, be greatest in Standard lead II; and examination of Standard lead II confirms this. The deflection in Standard lead II is upright and the axis must, therefore, be directed *towards the positive pole* of that lead.

The mean electrical axis is thus located parallel to the lead axis of Standard lead II and towards its positive pole. Reference to Figs. 108 and 109 shows that it is, therefore, located at +60°.

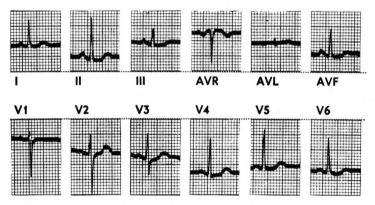

Fig. 112. Electrocardiogram: QRS axis directed to +60°; T wave axis directed to +30°; P wave axis directed to +60°.

(b) With reference to Fig. 79

The most equiphasic deflection in the six frontal plane leads is found in lead AVR. The mean manifest frontal plane axis thus runs at right angles to lead AVR. It is therefore, parallel to Standard lead III and the deflection must, therefore, be greatest in this lead; examination of Standard lead III confirms this. The deflection is upright or positive in Standard lead III and thus the mean axis is directed towards the positive pole of Standard lead III, i.e. it is located at +120°.

However, the deflection is not absolutely equiphasic in lead AVR, i.e. it is a little more positive than negative. Thus the axis is inclined a little towards the *positive pole of lead AVR* and is, therefore, located at about +130°.

Similarly, any electrocardiographic deflection may be expressed in terms of a mean manifest axis:

e.g. **The T Wave Axis:**
With reference to Fig. 112

1.   The most equiphasic T wave deflection is found in Standard lead III.
2.   The greatest T wave deflection is, consequently, found in lead AVR and is directed towards the negative pole of this lead.

The mean frontal plane T wave axis is thus located at +30°.

e.g. **The P Wave Axis:**
With reference to Fig. 112

1.   The most equiphasic P wave deflection is found in lead AVL.
2.   The greatest P wave deflection is, consequently, found in Standard lead II and is directed towards the positive pole of Standard lead II.

The mean frontal plane P wave axis is thus located at +60°.

The axes of some other electrocardiograms in this book are tabulated in Table 3.

AXIS DEVIATION

The normal range for the mean frontal plane QRS axis in the adult is **0° clockwise to +90°** (Fig. 108).

RIGHT AXIS DEVIATION

Right axis deviation is diagnosed when the axis is located in the range of **+90° clockwise to +180°** in the adult (Fig. 108).

The causes of right axis deviation

Right axis deviation may be associated with the following conditions:

Table 3. Table of electrical axes in some of the electrocardiograms in this book

	Mean Frontal Plane Axes		
	QRS	T	P
Fig. 19	+30°	+60°	+60°
Fig. 27B	+60°	−60°	+60°
Fig. 30	−50°	−40°	+60°
Fig. 32	+20°	0°	+50°
Fig. 36	−30°	−60°	+50°
Fig. 42	...	−50°	+60°
Fig. 43	+100°	+60°	+50°
Fig. 56	0°	+70°	+70°
Fig. 57	+60°	+100°	+60°
Fig. 58	+30°	+150°	+10°
Fig. 59	+50°	+40°	...
Fig. 68	+20°	...	+50°
Fig. 76	0°	−180°	+60°
Fig. 77	−20°	+50°	+50°
Fig. 79	+130°	0°	+50°
Fig. 80	+80°	0°	+70°
Fig. 91	+90°	+120°	...
Fig. 93	0°	+30°	+60°
Fig. 112	+60°	+30°	+60°
Fig. 152	+60°	+50°	−90°

1. *Right ventricular dominance.* See also Chapter 4, page 83.
2. *Reversed arm electrodes.* When the arm electrodes are reversed the mean manifest frontal plane QRS axis will be a mirror-image of the normal. And since the normal frontal plane QRS axis is usually directed at +60°, the axis with reversed arm electrodes will be directed at +120°. The precordial leads will reflect normal QRS patterns. Compare this with the manifestation of mirror-image dextrocardia where the precordial leads will reflect abnormal QRS patterns (see below).
3. *Mirror-image dextrocardia.* As with reversed arm electrodes this is also associated with a mean frontal plane QRS axis which is a mirror-image of the normal, i.e. an axis directed at +120°. In contrast to the manifestations resulting from reversed arm electrodes, however, the precordial leads will reflect tall R waves in leads V1 and V2 with progressive diminishing amplitude to lead V6.
4. *The Wolff-Parkinson-White syndrome.* The Wolff-Parkinson-White syndrome may be associated with a right axis deviation. The other features of this syndrome, viz. short P–R interval, delta wave

and secondary S-T segment and T wave changes make the diagnosis evident. See Chapter 21.

5. *Left posterior hemiblock.* This is associated with a right axis deviation but the diagnosis can only be established by exclusion of all the aforementioned causes of right axis deviation. See also page 120.

LEFT AXIS DEVIATION

Left axis deviation is diagnosed when the axis is in the range of 0° counter-clockwise to −120° (Fig. 109). This range has been arbitrarily sub-divided into slight left axis deviation: 0° to −29° and **significant left axis deviation: −30° to −120°.**

Mechanism and significance of left axis deviation

Axes between 0° and −29° were thought to be found occasionally in the normal subject, especially in those with obesity or a stocky build. It was also thought to be associated with ascites or other causes of abdominal distension such as pregnancy. Recent work, however (Schwartz & Schamroth, 1979)[8] has indicated that this is not so, since even the maximal distension of pregnancy is not associated with any form of left axis deviation; and may, at times, even be associated with some rightward deflection within the normal range. It now seems likely that axes within the zone of 0° to −29° are probably an expression of incomplete left anterior hemiblock.

Axes in the region of −30° to −120° nearly always connote organic heart disease. This is mainly due to **an intraventricular conduction defect involving the anterosuperior division of the left bundle branch:** a left anterior hemiblock (Grant 1956[2]; Davies & Evans, 1960[1]) (see below).

The causes of left axis deviation

Left axis deviation may be associated with the following conditions:

1. *Left anterior hemiblock.* Most cases of left axis deviation are very likely due to left anterior hemiblock. See below, page 119.

2. *Inferior wall myocardial infarction.* Inferior wall myocardial infarction is also associated with left axis deviation since the QRS forces are directed away from the inferior necrotic area, and thus upward and to the left. The associated clinical and other electrocardiographic features will establish the diagnosis.

3. *Emphysema—chronic obstructive airways disease.* Emphysema

may occasionally be associated with left axis deviation. The mechanism is uncertain.

4. *The Wolff-Parkinson-White syndrome.* The Wolff-Parkinson-White syndrome may be associated with a left axis deviation. The other features of this syndrome, viz. short P–R interval, delta wave and secondary S-T segment and T wave changes make the diagnosis evident. See chapter 21.

5. *An apical ectopic ventricular impulse.* An apical ectopic ventricular impulse such as the impulse of a ventricular extrasystole or a ventricular tachycardia may be associated with a left axis deviation.

6. *Apical pacing.* Electrical pacing from the apex of the heart may be associated with left axis deviation.

THE HEMIBLOCK CONCEPT

THE ANATOMY OF THE LEFT BUNDLE BRANCH SYSTEM

Shortly after leaving the main bundle of His, the left bundle branch divides into a number of rootlets, or fascicles, which then proceed in two major sweeps or radiations. These constitute the two major divisions or fascicles of the left bundle branch (Figs. 113 and 114).

The *anterosuperior division* which spreads anteriorly and superiorly over the subendocardium of the lateral wall of the left ventricle.

The *postero-inferior division* which spreads inferiorly and posteriorly over the diaphragmatic surface of the left ventricle.

The fibres of the two divisions meet and anastomose peripherally, forming a closed conduction network, a syncytium with rapid conduction properties.

The anterosuperior division of the left bundle branch is more vulnerable to disease processes than the postero-inferior division. This is because the anterosuperior division is relatively long and thin, whereas the postero-inferior division is relatively short and thick.[5] Furthermore, the postero-inferior division has a double blood supply in contrast to a single blood supply for the anterosuperior division.[6] The anterosuperior division is closer to the aortic valve, and is therefore more likely to be involved in disease processes affecting the aortic valve.[5] All these factors contribute to the greater vulnerability of the anterosuperior division.

Conduction within the left bundle branch system

Conduction through the anterosuperior division results in an activation front directed inferiorly and to the right (illustrated by Vector 2 in Fig. 113 and Vector 1 in Diagram A of Fig. 114). Conduction

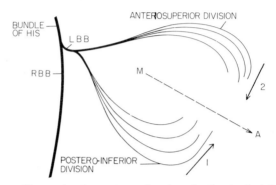

Fig. 113. Diagram illustrating the anatomy of, and conduction in, the left bundle branch. *Note*: The left bundle branch divides into two major sweeps or radiations—the anterosuperior division and the postero-inferior division. Conduction in the postero-inferior division is mainly upward and to the left; conduction in the anterosuperior division is mainly downward and to the right; simultaneous conduction through both divisions results in a mean axis—arrow labelled M-A—that is directed downward and to the left.

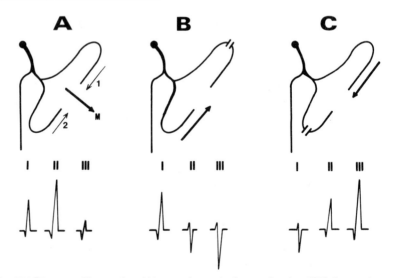

Fig. 114. Diagrams illustrating: (A) normal ventricular conduction, (B) left anterior hemiblock, and (C) left posterior hemiblock.

through the postero-inferior division results in an activation front directed *superiorly and to the left* (illustrated by Vector 1 in Fig. 113 and Vector 2 in Diagram A of Fig. 114). Since normal activation occurs concomitantly through both divisions, the two vectorial forces summate both complementing and modifying each other's direction and, thereby, resulting in a mean QRS force or vector which is directed downwards and to the left (illustrated by Vector M-A in Fig. 113 and Vector M in Diagram A of Fig. 114). This normal QRS axis is, therefore, commonly directed in the region of +60° on the frontal plane hexaxial reference system. The normal range for the mean frontal plane QRS axis in the adult is 0° to +90° (Fig. 108).

HEMIBLOCK

When conduction is delayed or interrupted in one of the divisions of the left bundle branch, it is termed a 'hemiblock'.[7]

LEFT ANTERIOR HEMIBLOCK

This results when conduction is interrupted in the anterosuperior division of the left bundle branch. When this occurs the activation front of the anterosuperior division is lost, i.e. Vector 1 in Diagram B of Fig. 114 is abolished. Activation now occurs predominantly through the fibres of the postero-inferior division. And since this activation front is directed upwards and to the left, the result is a *left axis deviation* (Diagram B of Fig. 114; Diagram A of Fig. 123). The resulting mean frontal plane QRS axis is commonly in the region of −30° counter-clockwise to −60°: the region of significant left axis deviation (Fig. 109). This will manifest empirically with deep terminal S waves in Standard leads II and III and lead AVF, and a tall R wave in lead AVL (Diagram B of Fig. 114 and Fig. 77).

Causes of left anterior hemiblock

Left anterior hemiblock may be due to the following causes:

Fibrosis and calcareous encroachment

Interruption of the anterosuperior division of the left bundle branch may be the result of fibrosis or calcareous encroachment from neighbouring structures (Diagram A in Fig. 123). This may be due to:
(i) the fibrosis resulting from chronic coronary insufficiency.

(ii) the fibrosis resulting from chronic cardiac failure.

(iii) the fibrosis resulting from chronic left ventricular decompensation in cases of systemic hypertension and other diseases associated with left ventricular failure. *Note.* Left ventricular hypertrophy *per se* does not cause left axis deviation; it is rather the associated fibrosis which is responsible (Grant, 1957[3]).

(iv) fibrosis associated with a chronic cardiomyopathy.

(v) calcareous encroachment on the left bundle branch conducting system from neighbouring structures such as the aortic valve and interventricular septum, also known as Lev's disease.[4]

(B) *Myocardial infarction*

Interruption of the anterosuperior division of the left bundle branch may be due to myocardial infarction. This results in *anterolateral peri-infarction block*. When this occurs, the initial vector is directed inferiorly and to the right, i.e. away from the infarcted anterolateral surface; an expression of the loss of forces due to the necrotic tissue itself. The terminal QRS forces are directed superiorly and to the left—the expression of the left anterior hemiblock (Diagram B of Fig. 123). See also section on Peri-infarction Block (page 128).

LEFT POSTERIOR HEMIBLOCK

This results when conduction is interrrupted in the postero-inferior division of the left bundle branch. When this occurs, the activation front of the postero-inferior division is lost, i.e. Vector 2 of Fig. 114 is abolished.

Activation now occurs predominantly through the fibres of the anterosuperior division (Diagram C of Fig. 114). And since this activation front is directed downwards and to the right, the result is a *right axis deviation* (Fig. 114C).

The mean manifest frontal plane QRS axis is rightwardly directed to the region of $+90°$ to $+120°$ on the hexaxial reference system (Vector 1 in Fig. 114). This results in prominent S waves in Standard lead I and lead AVL, and a tall R wave (of a qR complex) in Standard leads II, III and lead AVF (Fig. 115). The R wave is particularly tall in Standard lead III (Fig. 115). Note that this results in an S1, Q3, T3 manifestation, similar to that which occurs in acute pulmonary embolism (see page 85). Unlike acute pulmonary embolism, however, the amplitude of the deflections is not usually diminished, and may indeed be larger than normal (Fig. 115). Furthermore, unlike acute

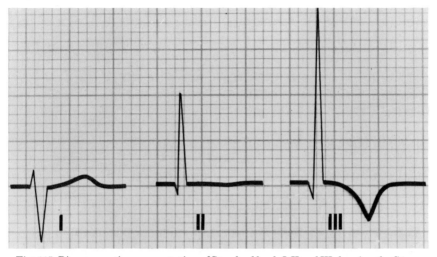

Fig. 115. Diagrammatic representation of Standard leads I, II and III showing the S1, Q3, T3 pattern of left posterior hemiblock.

pulmonary embolism, left posterior hemiblock is not necessarily associated with sinus tachycardia. Other causes of right axis deviation, such as right ventricular dominance, must be excluded on both clinical and electrocardiographic grounds before the diagnosis of right posterior hemiblock can be established. Left posterior hemiblock is consequently not a pure electrocardiographic diagnosis, but always a clinical-electrocardiographic correlation. See also section on Peri-infarction Block (page 128).

A 'NORTHWEST' QRS AXIS

A 'northwest' QRS axis—an axis directed to the region of −90° counterclockwise to −180°—may occur in the following circumstances:

1. *Marked right axis deviation.* This may occur, for example, with the marked right ventricular dominance associated with cyanotic congenital heart disease such as the Tetralogy of Fallot.

2. *Aneurysm of the left ventricular apex.* When an aneurysm involves the apex of the heart the effect is that of necrotic or inert tissue involving the apex of the heart. As indicated in Chapter 2, the QRS forces are directed away from inert or necrotic tissue. And since the apex of the heart is directed downwards and to the left, the QRS forces will be directed upwards and to the right—a 'northwest' axis.

3. *An apical ectopic ventricular impulse.* An apical ectopic ventricular impulse, such as the impulse of a ventricular extrasystole or
ventricular tachycardia, may be directed upwards and to the right.
4. *Apical pacing.* Electrical pacing from the apex of the heart may
be associated with a 'northwest' QRS axis.
5. The S1, S2, S3 syndrome (page 135) is, in effect, a 'northwest' axis
of the terminal QRS deflection.

FURTHER APPLICATION

SPECIFIC ORIENTATION OF THE LEAD AXES

Frontal and horizontal plane leads

The twelve conventional electrocardiographic leads may be divided
into two major groups on the basis of lead orientation (Fig. 115):
1. Standard leads I, II and III, and leads AVR, AVL and AVF are
orientated in the frontal plane and are termed the **frontal plane
leads.**
2. The precordial leads are orientated in the horizontal plane, i.e. at
right angles to the frontal plane leads, and are termed the **horizontal
plane leads.**

Leads orientated towards the cavity of the heart

Lead A VR: The positive pole of lead AVR is usually orientated to the
back of the atria and the cavities of the ventricles (Fig. 117). All
impulses are, therefore, directed away from the positive pole of lead
AVR; the P, QRS and T waves are, therefore, normally negative in
this lead. Diagnoses of abnormal electrocardiographic patterns must
only be based on positive deflections in this lead.

   Lead V1: Lead V1 is orientated to the proximal region of the free
wall of the right ventricle (Fig. 117). It therefore tends to be
orientated towards the base, or even the cavity, of the heart. And, as
with lead AVR, most deflections are, as a rule, predominantly
negative in this lead. Thus, generally speaking, diagnosis of abnormal electrocardiographic patterns is only based on positive deflections in this lead.

Leads orientated to the anterolateral surface of the heart (Figs. 12, 29 and 103)

Standard lead I.
Lead AVL.
Lateral precordial leads—leads V5 and V6.
Note. Lead V6—a horizontal plane lead—tends to be in the same plane as Standard lead I—a frontal plane lead (Fig. 116). Consequently, similar complexes are usually recorded by these leads.

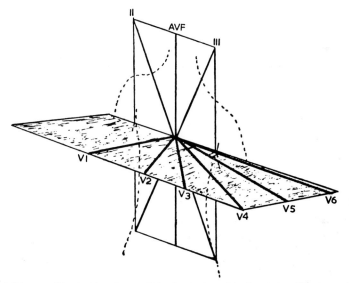

Fig. 116. Diagram illustrating the spatial orientation of the frontal and horizontal plane leads (see text).

Leads orientated to the inferior surface of the heart (Figs. 12, 37, 104 and 105)

Standard leads II and III.
Lead AVF.

Leads orientated to the anterior surface of the heart (Figs. 12 and 37)

Leads (V1) V2 to V6.

Leads orientated to the right ventricle (Fig. 33)

    Leads V1, V2 (V3).

Leads orientated to the left ventricle (Figs. 12 and 33)

    Leads (V4) V5 and V6.
    Standard lead I and lead AVL.

Leads orientated to the anteroseptal surface of the heart (Fig. 12)

    Leads V1 to V4.

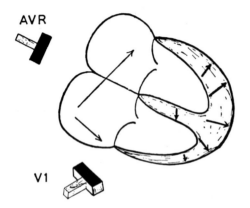

Fig. 117. Diagram illustrating the orientation of leads AVR and V1.

Leads usually reflecting the transition zone

    Usually leads V3 and V4.

Leads orientated towards the dominant ventricular muscle mass

      In the frontal plane: Standard lead II (Fig. 118).
      In the horizontal plane: usually lead V5 (Fig. 119).

THE QRS-T ANGLE

The mean frontal plane QRS axis and the mean frontal plane T wave axis are usually similarly directed, i.e. they are close to each other;

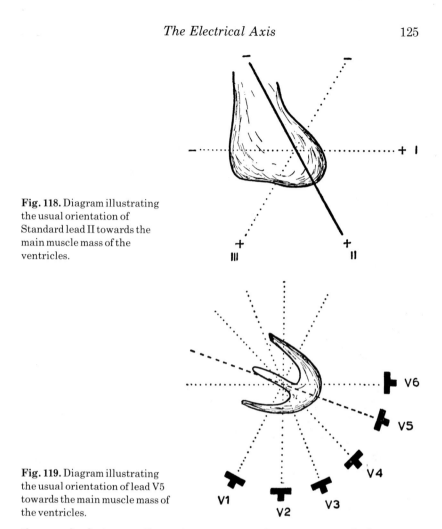

Fig. 118. Diagram illustrating the usual orientation of Standard lead II towards the main muscle mass of the ventricles.

Fig. 119. Diagram illustrating the usual orientation of lead V5 towards the main muscle mass of the ventricles.

the angle between them is consequently narrow and does not normally exceed 40°, and at most 60° (Fig. 120).

Myocardial ischaemia and the QRS-T angle

In the presence of myocardial disease—commonly myocardial ischaemia—the T wave axis tends to deviate from the diseased or ischaemic region whereas the QRS axis usually remains normally directed, or may even deviate in the opposite direction (Fig. 120). The angle between the QRS and T wave axes therefore widens, and it is usually a sign of myocardial disease when it exceeds 40°, or at most 60° in the adult.

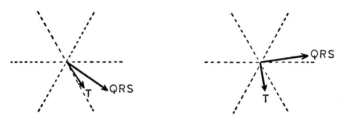

NORMAL   ISCHAEMIA

Fig. 120. Diagram illustrating the effect of myocardial ischaemia on the QRS-T angle. Normal: note the narrow QRS-T angle. Ischaemia: note the wide QRS-T angle as a result of a left anterior hemiblock.

Example I. The electrocardiogram shown in Fig. 112 has a normal QRS-T angle of 30° (QRS axis = +60°; T wave axis = +30°).

Example II. The electrocardiogram shown in Fig. 56 has a wide and abnormal QRS-T angle of 70° (QRS axis = 0°; T wave axis = +70°).

Note: This causes the T wave to be taller in Standard lead III than in Standard lead I.

The QRS-T angle is thus a sensitive index of significant T wave abnormality and is more reliable than the empirical observation of T wave change in isolated leads. Empirically, this may be expressed as follows: If the QRS complex is dominantly upright in Standard lead I, and the T wave is taller in Standard lead III than in Standard lead I, myocardial disease is usually present.

Hypertensive heart disease and the QRS-T angle

With hypertensive heart disease—left ventricular systolic over-load—the QRS axis is commonly directed at 0°, and the T wave axis is commonly directed diametrically opposite, at ±180° (Fig. 121). Empirically, this means that lead AVF will reflect an equiphasic QRS complex and an equiphasic T wave, whereas Standard lead I will reflect a dominantly upright QRS complex and an inverted T wave (Fig. 76).

Digitalis effect and the QRS-T angle

Therapeutic digitalis effect will diminish the magnitude of the T wave axis but will not change its direction. Digitalis toxicity, however, may rarely change the direction of the T wave axis. Thus, an abnormally wide QRS-T angle in a patient receiving digitalis

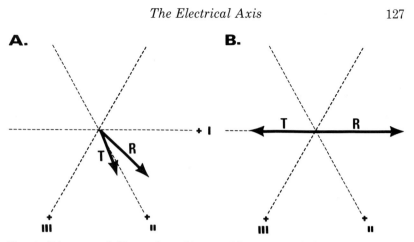

Fig. 121. Diagrammatic illustrations of A. normal frontal plane QRS and T wave axes, and B. frontal plane QRS and T wave axes commonly associated with left ventricular hypertrophy and strain—left ventricular systolic overload. Note (*a*) QRS axis is directed to 0°; (*b*) T wave axis is directed to ± 180°; (*c*) wide QRS-T angle of 180°.

indicates that the abnormality was present before the administration of the digitalis, or that the manifestation is a rare expression of digitalis toxicity.

The horizontal plane QRS-T angle

A wide QRS-T angle may also be reflected in the horizontal plane leads. The main horizontal plane QRS and T wave forces are normally directed towards lead V6 and away from lead V1 (Fig. 122). The QRS complex and T wave are, therefore, normally upright in lead V6 and negative in lead V1. Coronary insufficiency causes the T wave forces to deviate away from the QRS forces (Fig. 122). In the early stages of

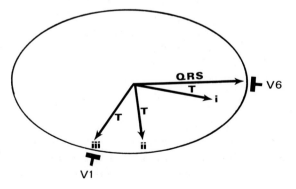

Fig. 122. Diagram illustrating the effects of coronary insufficiency on the horizontal plane QRS-T angle (see text).

this deviation (dotted arrows in Fig. 122), the T wave force may be more orientated towards lead V1 than lead V6 and the *T wave in lead V1 thus becomes taller than the T wave in lead V6*; the QRS complex remains directed to lead V6 which still records a tall R wave. This wide angle between the QRS and T wave forces in the horizontal plane—resulting in a *T-V1 taller than T-V6 syndrome*—may be the earliest sign of coronary insufficiency (see also page 54). Caution must, however, be exercised in the interpretation of the *T-V1 taller than T-V6 syndrome*, since errors in electrode placement can effect the same result. The QRS-T angle eventually becomes wider still and the T wave becomes frankly inverted in lead V6 and dominantly upright in lead V1.

The initial and terminal QRS forces

The mean QRS axis refers to the dominant, average or general direction of the QRS forces. Under certain circumstances, however, it is of value to consider the direction of the initial and terminal QRS forces separately. The direction of the first part of the QRS deflection is determined by only taking note of the first 0.04 sec of the QRS deflection in all the frontal plane leads, and ascertaining the direction of this initial vector in a manner similar to that used for the mean QRS axis (Grant, 1957[3]). The vector for the terminal 0.04 sec of the QRS deflection is similarly determined.

These initial and terminal forces may be compared with each other, as well as with the mean QRS axis. This may reveal such conditions as *peri-infarction block* and the S1, S2, S3 syndrome.

PERI-INFARCTION BLOCK AND THE VECTOR PRINCIPLES OF MYOCARDIAL INFARCTION

THE INITIAL 0.04 VECTOR

As indicated previously, the QRS forces are *directed away from the necrotic area of myocardial infarction* (see page 20 and Fig. 21). It is particularly the initial QRS forces that are directed away from the infarcted area, and leads orientated to this area will consequently record deep, wide pathological Q waves. Thus, a deep, wide Q wave is, in effect, a reflection of the initial 0.04 QRS vector being directed away from the positive pole of the lead. In inferior myocardial infarction, the initial QRS force moves away from the inferior or diaphragmatic surface of the heart, and leads orientated to this

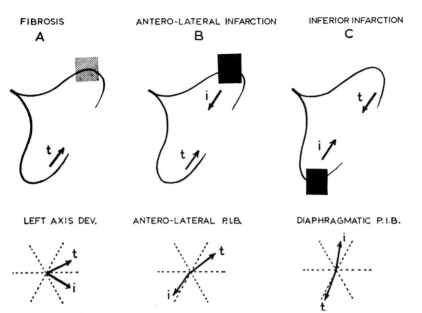

Fig. 123. Diagram illustrating the principles of (A) left axis deviation, (B) anterolateral peri-infarction block, (C) diaphragmatic peri-infarction block (see text).

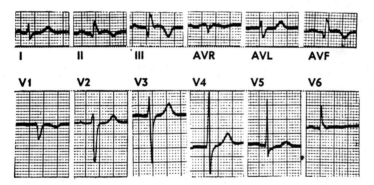

Fig. 124. Electrocardiogram illustrating acute inferolateral myocardial infarction with diaphragmatic peri-infarction block. Note pathological Q waves, raised convex-upward S-T segments and inverted T waves in Standard leads II and III, and lead AVF, and raised S-T segment and inverted T wave in lead V6, indicating inferolateral infarction. Initial QRS vector is located at $-60°$; the terminal QRS vector is located at $+120°$ (see text and Fig. 125).

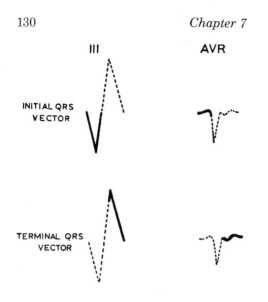

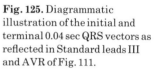

INITIAL QRS VECTOR

TERMINAL QRS VECTOR

Fig. 125. Diagrammatic illustration of the initial and terminal 0.04 sec QRS vectors as reflected in Standard leads III and AVR of Fig. 111.

surface (Standard leads II, III and lead AVF) will reflect deep, wide Q waves. Viewed vectorially, the initial vector will be located in the region of $-60°$ to $-100°$ on the hexaxial reference system (vector i in Diagram C of Fig. 123).

Example I. With reference to Fig. 124. When only the initial 0.04 part of the QRS deflection is considered, the largest deflection occurs in Standard lead III and is negative in this lead (Fig. 124); the initial 0.04 part of the QRS complex is almost equiphasic in lead AVR. See also Fig. 125. The initial vector is thus located at $-60°$, i.e. away from the inferior wall of the ventricles.

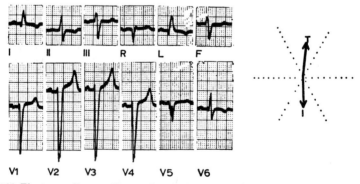

Fig. 126. Electrocardiogram illustrating the features of anterolateral peri-infarction block. Initial vector (labelled I) located at $+90°$ on the hexaxial reference system. Terminal vector (labelled T) located at $-80°$ on the hexaxial reference system (see text).

Example II. With reference to Fig. 126. When only the initial 0.04 part of the QRS deflection is considered, the largest deflection occurs in lead AVF and is positive in this lead; the initial 0.04 part of the QRS complex is equiphasic in Standard lead I. The initial vector is thus located at $+90°$.

THE TERMINAL 0.04 VECTOR

As indicated previously, the left bundle branch divides into two major sweeps or radiations: the anterosuperior division and the postero-inferior division (Figs. 113, 114, 123). If conduction is interrupted in the branches of the anterosuperior division (Fig. 114 and Diagrams A and B of Fig. 123) activation of the ventricles will be effected principally through the branches of the postero-inferior division; the vector will therefore be directed upwards and to the left. This deviation affects principally the terminal 0.04 vector, i.e. there is a terminal left axis deviation. This type of interruption may be due to *fibrosis* or *infarction* involving the anterolateral aspect of the left ventricle. It will be noted that, in the case of infarction, the *terminal vector points towards the infarcted area.*

If conduction is interrupted in the branches of the postero-inferior division of the left bundle branch, activation of the ventricles will be effected principally through the branches of the anterosuperior division; the terminal vector will then be directed downwards and to the right (vector t in Diagram C of Fig. 123), i.e. there is a terminal right axis deviation.

Interruption of the postero-inferior division is mainly due to inferior myocardial infarction, and it is noteworthy that the *terminal vector is again directed towards the infarcted area.*

Example I. With reference to Fig. 124. The largest deflection of the terminal 0.04 sec of the QRS complex occurs in Standard lead III and is positive in this lead; the most equiphasic deflection of the terminal 0.04 sec of the QRS complex occurs in lead AVR. The terminal 0.04 sec vector is, therefore, located at $+120°$. These principles are diagrammatically illustrated in Diagram C of Fig. 123 and Fig. 125.

Summary of QRS vectors in Fig. 124

    Initial 0.04 sec QRS vector located at $-60°$.
    Terminal 0.04 sec QRS vector located at $+120°$.
    Angle between initial and terminal 0.04 sec QRS vectors: $180°$.

Example II. With reference to Fig. 126. The largest deflection of the terminal 0.04 sec of the QRS complex occurs in lead AVF and is negative in this lead; the most equiphasic deflection occurs in Standard lead I (it is slightly more positive than negative). The terminal vector is therefore located at $-80°$.

Summary of QRS vectors in Fig. 126

>Initial 0.04 sec QRS vector located at $+90°$.
>Terminal 0.04 sec QRS vector located at $-80°$.
>Angle between initial terminal 0.04 sec QRS vectors: 170°.

On the basis of the aforementioned principles, it will be noted that (*a*) the initial 0.04 QRS vector is directed *away* from the infarcted area, and (*b*) when the infarct interrupts either the anterosuperior or postero-inferior divisions of the left bundle branch, the terminal 0.04 sec QRS vector is directed *towards* the infarcted area. This will result in a *wide angle—greater than* 100°—*between the initial and terminal QRS vectors* and is termed **peri-infarction block.**

When an anterolateral infarction interrupts the anterosuperior division of the left bundle branch, the initial vector is directed downwards and to the right, and the terminal vector is directed upwards and to the left (Diagram B of Fig. 123). This is termed **anterolateral peri-infarction block.**

When an inferior infarction interrupts the postero-inferior division of the left bundle branch, the initial vector is directed upwards and to the left, and the terminal vector is directed downwards and to the right (Diagram C of Fig. 123). This is termed **diaphragmatic peri-infarction block.**

Note. When left axis deviation is due to fibrosis only, the angle between the initial and terminal QRS forces is narrow.

Summary of the vector principles in myocardial infarction (Fig. 127)

1. The initial QRS vector is directed away from the infarcted area (vector 1 in Fig. 127). This results in a deep, wide, initial pathological Q wave or a QS complex in leads directed towards the infarcted area.
2. The terminal QRS vector is directed towards the infarcted area (vector 2 in Fig. 127). This only occurs in some cases of anterolateral and inferior myocardial infarctions.
3. The S-T segment vector is directed towards the surface of the

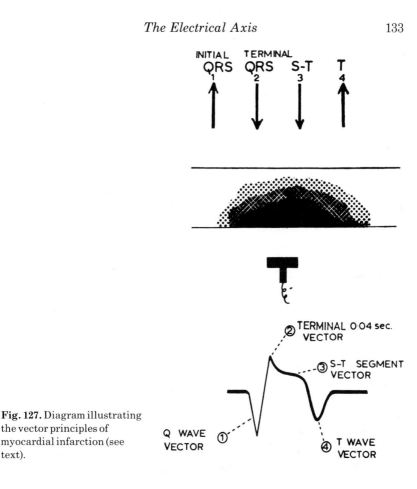

Fig. 127. Diagram illustrating the vector principles of myocardial infarction (see text).

injured zone of the infarcted area (vector 3 in Fig. 127). This results in a raised S-T segment in leads orientated towards the infarcted area.
4.   The T wave vector is directed away from the ischaemic zone of the infarcted area (vector 4 in Fig. 127). This results in an inverted T wave in leads orientated towards the infarcted area.

The vectorial significance of a Q wave in Standard lead III

A Q wave of a Qr complex in Standard lead III is often a sign of old inferior myocardial infarction. However, a Q wave in this lead may also occur normally. Vectorial evaluation will assist in the differentiation.

A Q wave will appear in Standard lead III if the initial vector is situated anywhere in the hemisphere between +30° counter-clockwise to $-150°$ on the hexaxial reference system. When this occurs, the initial vector will always be orientated towards the negative pole of the Standard lead III lead axis, since this is the negative zone for Standard lead III.

When the initial QRS vector is situated in the region of $0°$ to $+30°$, a Q wave will appear in Standard lead III *only*, i.e. there will be no Q waves in lead AVF or Standard lead II as the vector is directed towards the positive poles of these leads, i.e. it is still within the positive zone of these leads (Diagram A of Fig. 128). This vector is directed laterally and to the left, i.e. it is not directed away from the inferior wall of the ventricle and is, therefore, not likely to be significant of myocardial infarction. In other words, a Q wave which appears in Standard lead III only is unlikely to be an expression of myocardial infarction.

When the initial QRS vector is situated in the region $0°$ to $-30°$ (Diagram B of Fig. 128) it is directed towards the negative poles of Standard lead III *and* lead AVF, and a Q wave will be recorded by both these leads. This initial vector is directed laterally and to the left, i.e. it is still *not* directed away from the inferior wall of the ventricle, and is therefore also not likely to be significant of inferior myocardial infarction.

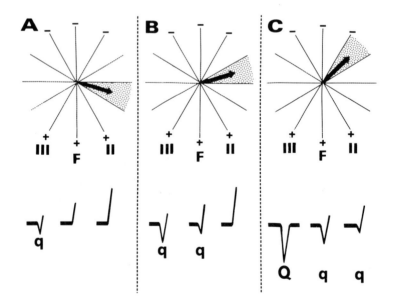

Fig. 128. Diagrams illustrating the vectorial significance of a Q wave in Standard lead III.

When the initial QRS vector is situated in the region of $-30°$ counter-clockwise to $-150°$ (Diagram C of Fig. 128) it is directed towards the negative poles of Standard leads II and III, and lead AVF, and a Q wave will appear in all these leads. Furthermore, the initial QRS vector is now directed superiorly, i.e. away from the inferior wall of the ventricle and may thus be indicative of inferior myocardial infarction.

Thus, a Q wave in Standard lead III is significant of inferior myocardial infarction under the following circumstances:

(*a*) When it fulfils the criteria of size and duration for a pathological Q wave (page 41).

(*b*) When it is *associated with a prominent Q wave in lead AVF, and a prominent or at the very least a normal q wave in Standard lead II*. In other words, the diagnosis of inferior wall myocardial infarction cannot be entertained if there is no q wave in Standard lead II.

Note. Marked left axis deviation of the mean QRS axis, e.g. $-70°$, will result in dominantly negative deflections in Standard leads II and III, and lead AVF, which may, at times, mimic pathological Q waves.

The S1, S2, S3 syndrome

This syndrome is characterized by a terminal QRS vector that is directed *superiorly and to the right*, i.e. a vector located in the region of $-90°$ counter-clockwise to $-150°$ on the hexaxial system (Fig. 129). This vector is in the area of negativity for all the Standard leads and will thus produce prominent S waves in all the Standard leads (Fig. 130). The mean QRS axis is usually normal in direction.

This syndrome may be found in the following conditions (Grant, 1957[3]):

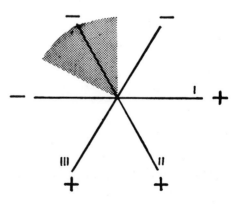

Fig. 129. The hexaxial reference system. The shaded area denotes the region of negativity for all three Standard leads, i.e. the location of the terminal QRS vector in the S1, S2, S3 syndrome.

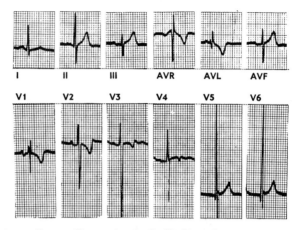

Fig. 130. Electrocardiogram illustrating the S1, S2, S3 syndrome.

1. It may be **normal,** and probably represents persistence of the juvenile pattern of right ventricular dominance (see below).

2. It may be associated with **right ventricular hypertrophy** and is believed to represent hypertrophy of the right ventricular outflow tract—the *crista supraventricularis. Note:* the S1, S2, S3 syndrome constitutes supportive but not diagnostic evidence of right ventricular hypertrophy.

3. It may occasionally be associated with **myocardial infarction;** there will, however, always be other evidence of myocardial infarction, i.e. deformity of the initial QRS vector and/or S-T segment and T wave changes.

THE P WAVE AXIS

The normal P wave axis

The normal P wave axis is usually directed in the region of $+40°$ to $+60°$ on the frontal plane hexaxial reference system (Region E of Fig. 131).

The abnormal P wave axis

RIGHT ATRIAL ENLARGEMENT

P. pulmonale and P. congenitale

Right atrial enlargement is associated with a tall peaked P wave in Standard lead II (page 102). This form of P wave may be found in

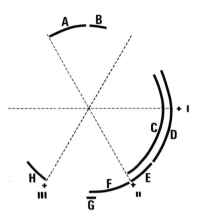

Fig. 131. Diagrammatic representation illustrating the distribution of various forms of frontal plane P wave axes (see text).

association with either acquired or congenital heart disease. The P wave associated with each condition may be differentiated on a vectorial basis as follows (Sodi-Pallares & Calder, 1956[9]):

P. pulmonale. When P wave enlargement is associated with acquired heart disease, the P wave vector is usually directed in the region of + 60° to + 90° on the hexaxial reference system (Region F of Fig. 131). When the acquired heart disease is emphysema, the P wave axis is usually in the region of + 90° (Region G of Fig. 131).

P. congenitale. When P wave enlargement is associated with congenital heart disease, the P wave vector is usually directed in the region of − 30° clockwise to + 60° on the hexaxial reference system, i.e. the P wave axis rarely deviates further to the right than + 60° (Region C of Fig. 131).

LEFT ATRAL ENLARGEMENT

With left atrial enlargement the P wave axis tends to deviate to the left and may be situated in the region of + 40° counter-clockwise to − 30° (Region D of Fig. 131).

The P wave axis of retrograde atrial activation

Retrograde activation of the atria is directed cranially, and is thus associated with a superiorly directed P′ wave axis, i.e. an axis in the region of − 80° to − 100° (Regions A and B of Fig. 131). With retrograde atrial activation associated with impulses of A-V nodal or ventricular origin, the P′ wave axis is usually directed to the region of − 80° to − 90° on the frontal hexaxial reference system. It rarely is further to the left than $-90°$. Thus, the P′ wave of A-V nodal rhythms of that of impulses passing through the A-V node will be negative in Standard leads II and III, and lead AVF, but equiphasic in Standard lead I. Retrograde atrial activation may also be associated with reciprocal rhythm of atrial origin where the sinus impulse after its passage through the A-V node enters an A-V junctional by-pass—the Kent bundle—and returns retrogradely to activate the atria a second time. When this occurs, the P′ wave axis is directed superiorly and to the region of $-90°$ to $-100°$ (Region A of Fig. 131). This means that the P wave will be negative in Standard lead II and III, lead AVF as well as in Standard lead I.

'Mirror-image' dextrocardia

In 'mirror-image' dextrocardia, the P wave axis is directed to the right, in the region of $+120°$ to $+150°$ (Region H of Fig. 131). A similar P wave axis will occur when the right and left arm electrodes are reversed.

REFERENCES

1 DAVIES J. N. P. & EVANS W. (1960) The significance of deep S waves in leads II and III. *Brit. Heart J.* **22,** 55.
2 GRANT R. P. (1956) Left axis deviation. *Circulation* **14,** 233.
3 GRANT R. P. (1957) *Clinical Electrocardiography.* New York: McGraw-Hill.
4 LEV M. (1964) Anatomic basis for atrioventricular block. *Amer. J. Med.* **37,** 742.
5 ROSENBACH M. B. (1968) Types of right bundle branch block and their clinical significance. *J. Electrocardiol.* **1,** 221.
6 ROSENBAUM M. B. (1970) In *Symposium on Cardiac Arrhythmias,* ed. Sandoe E., Flensted-Jensen E. & Olesen K. H. Sodertalje, Sweden: A. B. Astra.
7 ROSENBAUM M. B., ELIZARI M. V. & LAZZARI J. O. (1970) *The Hemiblocks.* Oldsmar, Florida: Tampa Tracings.
8 SCHWARTZ D. B. & SCHAMROTH L. (1979) Effect of pregnancy on the frontal plane QRS axis. *J. Electrocardiol.* **12,** 279.
9 SODI-PALLARES D. & CALDER R. M. (1956) *New Bases of Electrocardiography.* St. Louis, Illinois: C. V. Mosby Company.

Chapter 8
Hypothermia

Hypothermia manifests electrocardiographically as follows (illustrated in Fig. 132):

1. *Sinus bradycardia.* The result of a profound depression of pacemaker automaticity.

2. *Muscle tremor—'shivering'—artifact.*

3. *J wave.* This is a rounded, rather narrow, 'hump-like' wave usually superimposed on the distal limb of the QRS complex, and thought to be due to early repolarization. This is also known as the Osborne wave.

4. *Prolonged Q-T interval.*

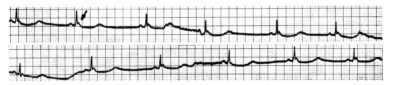

Fig. 132. Electrocardiogram (continuous strip of Standard lead II) showing the features of hypothermia. *Note*: 1. sinus bradycardia. 2. The *J* wave (example illustrated with arrow). 3. 'Shivering'—muscle tremor—artifact. 4. Prolonged Q–T interval. The Q–Tc is 0.58 sec.

Chapter 9
Electrical Alternans

Electrical alternans is an electrocardiographic manifestation in which there is alternation in the amplitude of the QRS complexes and/or the T waves (Fig. 133). It often accompanies fast rates and then has no prognostic significance. When found with slow rates it has the same significance as its mechanical counterpart and usually connotes organic heart disease with an adverse prognosis. Electrical alternans may occasionally be associated with a pericardial effusion.[1] When this occurs, the alternans is usually best seen in the mid-precordial leads.

Note: Electrical alternans does not cause a disturbance of rhythm.

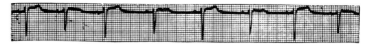

Fig. 133. Electrocardiogram (Standard lead III) showing electrical alternans. Note (*a*) the alternation in the amplitude of the QRS complexes and T waves; (*b*) there is no disturbance of rhythm. This electrical alternans is significant of myocardial disease since it occurs with a relatively slow heart rate.

REFERENCE

1 McGregor M. & Baskind E. (1955) Electrical alternans in pericardial effusion. *Circulation* **11,** 837.

Chapter 10
The Q–T Interval

The Q–T interval is the interval from the *beginning* of the QRS complex to the *end* of the T wave. It represents the total duration of the electrical activity of the ventricles, viz. the sum of ventricular depolarization and repolarization.

Measurement of the Q–T interval

Measurement of the Q–T interval may, on occasion, present some difficulty since the exact beginning and end of the interval may be difficult to determine. The beginning of the QRS complex is best, and should preferably be determined in a lead showing a QRS complex with an initial q wave—commonly Standard leads I or II, and leads AVL, V5 and V6. This is necessary in order to avoid the mistake of ignoring an initial part of the QRS complex which may be isoelectric in a particular lead and hence not discernible; the q wave being, in effect, incorporated within the P–R interval. If cognizance is not taken of this, an unduly and incorrectly short interval may be measured.

Determining the precise end of the Q–T interval may, at times, also present some difficulty. This is because the end of the T wave may be obscured by a superimposed U wave or, in the case of sinus tachycardia, by the ensuing P wave. The U wave deflection is usually minimal or isoelectric in lead AVL. This is because the U wave axis is usually directed at +60° on the frontal plane. It is, therefore, perpendicular or at right-angles to the lead axis of lead AVL and will consequently make a minimal, equiphasic or isoelectric lead from which to measure the Q–T interval, since the end of the T wave is least likely to be obscured by a U wave.

When the Q–T interval is measured from a lead where the U wave is prominent, the dip or notch between the T and U waves is taken as the end of the T wave. This is not necessarily the true end-point of the T wave, but it will do for practical purposes. The Q–T interval varies with age, sex and heart rate.

141

THE SIGNIFICANCE OF HEART RATE IN RELATIONSHIP TO THE Q–T INTERVAL

The Q–T interval shortens with tachycardia and lengthens with bradycardia[7, 11] In other words, the Q–T interval shortens with a diminution of the R–R interval and lengthens with an increase of the R–R interval. This is due almost solely to a shortening or lengthening of the myocardial refractory period—a shortening or lengthening of ventricular repolarization. It is thus evident that, for a meaningful evaluation, the Q–T interval cannot be viewed in absolute terms but must be corrected for the effect of the associated sinus rate.

THE CORRECTED Q–T INTERVAL: THE Q–TC

Calculation of the Q–Tc. The Q–T interval is corrected for what it would theoretically be at a rate of 60 beats per minute. The corrected Q–T interval is known as the Q–Tc. Various formulae have been proposed for correction of the Q–T interval. The most frequently used is that propounded by Bazett.[3] Bazett's formula states:

$$Q–Tc = \frac{Q–T}{\sqrt{R–R}}$$

The Q–T interval is measured as described. The R–R interval is measured between two consecutive R waves. Both figures are expressed in seconds. The Q–Tc may be regarded as a constant—K. Thus:

$$K = \frac{Q–T}{\sqrt{R–R}}$$

The normal value for K is 0.39 sec $\pm$ 0.04 sec. The normal range is thus from 0.35 to 0.43 sec.[6]

The value of the Q–Tc or K corresponds to the Q–T duration at a heart rate of 60 per minute. For, at this rate, the R–R interval is 1.0 sec, and since the square root of 1.0 sec is still 1.0 sec, the Q–T will be constant.

COMMENTS

1. When the rhythm is irregular, as is marked sinus arrhythmia or atrial fibrillation, the mean R–R interval and mean Q–T interval of at least 10 beats must be determined.

2. In hypokalaemia the T wave becomes low to inverted and may even disappear. The U wave becomes taller and very prominent. When this occurs the U wave may be mistaken for the T wave and a false prolongation of the Q–T interval diagnosed (Figs. 90, 91 and 92).

Causes of prolonged Q–Tc

A long Q–Tc may be associated with the following conditions:

(*a*) Hypocalcaemia[2]: The prolongation of the Q–Tc in this condition is due mainly to a prolongation of the S–T segment. The T wave remains normal (page 98, Fig. 94).

(*b*) Acute Rheumatic Carditis[1, 4, 10, 13]: note that although the presence of a prolonged Q–Tc is evidence of acute carditis, a normal Q–Tc does not exclude the diagnosis.

(*c*) Acute myocardial infarction.[9]

(*d*) Acute myocarditis of any cause.

(*e*) Quinidine effect.[12]

(*f*) Procaine amide effect.

(*g*) Sympathetic stimulation, as may be associated with a head injury, cerebral haemorrhage or a syncopal attack (see page 213, Fig. 184).

(*h*) Hypothermia (page 139, Fig. 132).

Causes of a short Q–Tc

A short Q–Tc may be associated with the following conditions:

Digitalis effect[5] (page 93).

Hypercalcaemia[8] (page 100, Fig. 95).

Hyperthermia.

Vagal stimulation.

REFERENCES

1 ABRAHAMS D. G. (1949) The QT interval in acute rheumatic carditis. *Brit. Heart J.* **11**, 342.

2 BARKER P. S., JOHNSON F. D. & WILSON F. N. (1937) The duration of systole in hypocalcemia. *Am. Heart J.* **14**, 82.

3 BAZETT H. O. (1918–20) An analysis of the time relations of electrocardiograms. *Heart* **7**, 353.

4 EPSTEIN N. A. (1950) A study of the QTc in the electrocardiogram in rheumatic fever. *J. Pediat.* **36**, 583.

5 GOLDBERGER E. (1944) Studies on unipolar leads. IV. The effects of Digitalis. *Am. Heart J.* **28**, 370.

6 HEGGLIN R. & HOLZMANN M. (1937) QT-Dauer. *Z. klin. Med.* **132,** 1.
7 HORWITZ O. & GRAYBIEL A. (1948) Prolongation of the Q–T interval in the electrocardiogram occurring as a temporary functional disturbance in healthy persons. *Am. Heart J.* **35,** 480.
8 KELLOG F. & KERR W.J. (1936) Electrocardiographic changes in hyperparathyroidism. *Am. Heart J.* **12,** 346.
9 KRASNOFF S. O. (1950) The duration of the Q–T interval in myocardial infarction. *Am. Heart J.* **39,** 523.
10 POKRESS M. & GOLDBERGER E. (1949) A study of the Q–T interval in rheumatic fever. *Am. Heart J.* **38,** 423.
11 ROBB J. S. & TURMAN W. G. (1947) Further consideration of the QT interval. *Am. J. Med. Sci.* **214,** 180.
12 SAGALL E.L., HORN C.D. & RISEMAN J. E. F. (1943) Studies on the activity of Quinidine in man. *Arch. Int. Med.* **71,** 460.
13 TARAN L. M. & SZILAGYI N. (1947) The duration of the electrical systole (Q–T) in acute rheumatic carditis in children. *Am. Heart J.* **33,** 14.

PART II
DISORDERS OF CARDIAC RHYTHM

SECTION 1: Basic Principles
SECTION 2: Disorders of Impulse Formation
SECTION 3: Disorders of Impulse Conduction
SECTION 4: The Secondary Disorders of Rhythm
SECTION 5: Correlative Essay—Structural Nodal disease

SECTION 1
BASIC PRINCIPLES

Chapter 11
Basic Principles

The electrocardiogram is conventionally recorded at a speed of 25 mm per second. The electrocardiographic paper is divided into large and small squares (Fig. 134).

Each large square represents 0.20 sec.

Five large squares represent 1 sec.

Fifteen large squares represent 3 sec.

Each small square represents 0.04 ($\frac{1}{25}$) sec.

Note: Most recording graphs have every fifteenth large square marked by a vertical line on the upper border of the recording paper (Fig. 137)

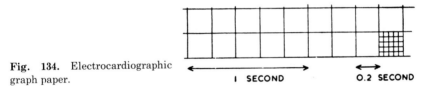

Fig. 134. Electrocardiographic graph paper.

I SECOND   0.2 SECOND

The cardiac rate may be estimated by counting the number of cardiac cycles—R–R intervals—in fifteen squares (3 sec) and multiplying by 20, or the number of cycles in 6 sec (the interval between two vertical lines on the upper border of the recording paper), and multiplying this by ten. The cardiac rate may also be calculated by dividing the figure of 6000 by the R–R interval (in hundredths of a sec). For example, the R–R interval in Fig. 137 measures 1.44 sec. Therefore the rate is $6000 \div 144 = 42$ per minute.

ANATOMY AND PHYSIOLOGY OF THE CONDUCTING SYSTEM

The rate and rhythm of the heart are controlled by the **sino-atrial**

147

node (S-A node), which is situated in the wall of the right atrium to the right of the superior vena caval orifice (Fig. 2). The sinus impulse leaves the S-A node and spreads through the atrial muscle; this atrial activation is reflected by the P wave of the electrocardiogram. The sinus impulse eventually reaches the A-V node which is situated in the right atrium above the tricuspid valve and just to the right of the interatrial septum. After a delay at the A-V node (reflected in the electrocardiogram as the greater part of the P–R interval) the impulse travels down the bundle of His, bundle branches and Purkinje network system. The **bundle of His** passes horizontally to the left from the A-V node, pierces the membranous interventricular septum and divides into **right and left bundle branches**. These pass down on either side of the muscular interventricular septum and finally divide into the **Purkinje network of fibres** which proceed vertically to the surface of the heart from the endocardium to the epicardium (see also page 5 and Figs. 2 and 4).

The S-A node is mainly under the influence of the vagus nerve and normal variations in heart rate are effected mainly by variations in vagal tone. An *increase* in vagal tone slows the heart; a *decrease* in vagal tone accelerates the heart. The S-A node is also influenced to a lesser degree by variations in sympathetic tone.

The pacemakers of the heart

The heart has many potential pacemaking cells. These are situated in the S-A node, the A-V node, the bundle of His, the atria, and the ventricles (every Purkinje cell is a potential pacemaking cell). The S-A node has the fastest inherent discharge rate which usually ranges from 70 to 80 beats per minute. The inherent rate of potential A-V nodal pacemaking cells is about 60 beats per minute. The inherent rate of pacemaking cells in the bundle of His is about 50 beats per minute. The inherent rate of the Purkinje cells of the ventricular muscle is about 30 to 40 beats per minute. In other words, the more distal a potential pacemaker is situated from the S-A node, the slower its inherent discharge rate.

There is, however, only one pacemaker that is normally in the control of the heart. This is the S-A node, the pacemaker with the fastest inherent discharge rate. Its impulse reaches the slower subsidiary pacemakers before they have an opportunity to mature and 'fire' spontaneously, and discharges them prematurely. Thus, the slower potential pacemaking cells enjoy *no protection* from the impulses of the fastest pacemaker.

CLASSIFICATION OF THE ARRHYTHMIAS

Abnormal rhythms occur as primary and secondary disorders. Primary disorders of rhythm reflect a basic, essential abnormality.

Secondary disorders of rhythm only occur as a result of, and secondary to, a primary disorder.

The primary disorders of rhythm

The primary disorders of rhythm may, in simplified form, be classified into two major categories:
1. Disturbances of impulse formation, and
2. Disturbances of impulse conduction.

1. DISTURBANCES OF IMPULSE FORMATION

Sinus rhythms

Sinus arrhythmia
Sinus tachycardia
Sinus bradycardia

Ectopic atrial rhythms

Atrial extrasystoles
Paroxysmal atrial tachycardia
Atrial fibrillation
Atrial flutter

A-V nodal rhythms

A-V nodal extrasystoles
Extrasystolic—paroxysmal—A-V nodal tachycardia
Idionodal tachycardia

Ventricular rhythms

Ventricular extrasystoles
Extrasystolic ventricular tachycardia
Idioventricular tachycardia
Ventricular flutter

Ventricular fibrillation
Ventricular parasystole

2. DISTURBANCES OF IMPULSE CONDUCTION

S-A block
A-V block
The Wolff-Parkinson-White Syndrome
Reciprocal rhythms

The secondary disorders of rhythm

Escape rhythms
     Atrial escape
     A-V nodal escape
     Ventricular escape
A-V dissociation
Phasic aberrant ventricular conduction

THE DIAGNOSTIC APPROACH TO ABNORMAL HEART RHYTHMS

FUNDAMENTAL DESCRIPTIVE PROPERTIES OF CARDIAC RHYTHMS

There are three fundamental aspects to every cardiac rhythm:

1. *The rhythm has an anatomical origin*: the impulse may arise in the sino-atrial node, the atria, the A-V node and the ventricles.
2. *The rhythm has a discharge sequence*: normal inherent discharge, (as would occur in normal sinus rhythm or an idioventricular escape rhythm), tachycardia, bradycardia, extrasystole, parasystole, flutter or fibrillation.
3. *The rhythm has a conduction sequence*: for example, 2:1 A-V block, complete A-V block, 2:1 S-A block.

Any description of a cardiac rhythm is incomplete without reference to all three of these fundamental aspects. This principle is all too frequently ignored. For example, the statement is often made that the patient has 'second degree A-V block'. This statement is incomplete and has relatively little meaning. Thus, a 2:1 A-V block may complicate an atrial flutter with a rate of 300 per minute. The block, under these circumstances, is a physiological phenomenon, and does not imply an increase in refractoriness or disease of the A-V conducting tissues. A 2:1 A-V block may also complicate normal sinus rhythm with a rate of 65 per minute. Under these circum-stances, the block usually connotes an absolute increase in refractor-iness, and is most commonly an expression of some disease state of the A-V conducting tissues. The unqualified diagnosis of second degree A-V block is therefore incomplete, too broad in concept and may in fact be misleading. Similarly, an unqualified statement of the discharge sequence—tachycardia, flutter, fibrillation, etc.—is obviously meaningless without a qualification of the impulse origin. Clearly then, the most important single aspect of any arrhythmia is its anatomical site of origin—S-A node, atria, A-V node or ventricles. It must, however, be stressed that all three aspects of the arrhythmia must be stated. For example, the diagnosis of 'atrial flutter' is frequently not qualified any further. However, from a haemodynamic and clinical viewpoint, it is of the utmost importance to know whether the atrial flutter is conducted with a 1:1 A-V conduction—resulting in a rapid ventricular rate and haemodynamic embarrass-ment, or, 4:1 A-V conduction resulting in a slow ventricular rate with minimal haemodynamic embarrassment. Similarly, the diagnosis of 'normal sinus rhythm' is incomplete unless the conduction sequence is stated. Although the unqualified statement of 'normal sinus rhythm' is often meant to imply normal conduction to the ventricles, this is not necessarily so. Normal sinus rhythm may, for example, be complicated by complete A-V block.

THE DESCRIPTION OF DUAL RHYTHMS

A dual rhythm is a rhythm wherein two pacemakers concomitantly contribute to the rhythm of the heart. A dual rhythm is present in every form of A-V dissociation—one pacemaker activating the atria and the other the ventricles. When this occurs, the descriptive properties of both the dissociated rhythms must be stated.

Examples
   (a) *Sinus rhythm* with complete A-V block and an *idioventricular escape rhythm.*
   (b) *Ventricular tachycardia* with A-V nodal interference dissocia-tion from *normal sinus rhythm.*

The basic approach

On the basis of the aforementioned principles cardiac rhythm may be fundamentally analysed as follows.

1. The atrial deflection is defined and analysed to determine whether it represents:
    (*a*) a normal *P* wave
    (*b*) an ectopic or *P'* deflection
    (*c*) a flutter—*F*—wave
    (*d*) a chaotic fibrillation—*f*—wave.
2. The atrial rate is determined.
3. The regularity of the atrial rhythm is determined.
4. The relationship of the atrial deflections to the QRS complexes is determined.
5. The QRS configuration is analysed.

THE GRAPHIC REPRESENTATION OF INTRACARDIAC CONDUCTION

Intracardiac conduction may be conveniently and conventionally represented by means of a 'ladder' diagram. This is a graphic representation: the ordinate represents the anatomic levels of S-A node, atria, A-V node and ventricles; the abscissa represents time (Fig. 135).

Diagram A of Fig. 135 illustrates normal conduction of a sinus impulse. The impulse—black dot—arises in the sino-atrial node (S-A) and is conducted relatively quickly through the atria (A) as reflected by the relatively steep slope. The impulse is delayed within the A-V node or junction (A-V) as reflected by the relatively gradual slope, and is finally conducted relatively quickly through the ventricles (V) as reflected once again by a relatively steep slope.

Diagram B of Fig. 135 represents first degree A-V block—a prolonged P–R interval—a delay in conduction through the A-V

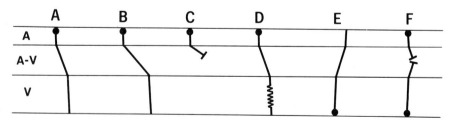

Fig. 135. Graphic representation of the use of the 'ladder' diagram in depicting arrhythmias. The ordinate reflects the anatomical levels. The abscissa reflects time. The black dot reflects impulse origin. A = normal conduction. B = delayed A-V conduction. C = A-V block. D = aberrant ventricular conduction. E = ectopic ventricular impulse with retrograde A-V conduction to the atria. F = interference between a sinus impulse and an ectopic ventricular impulse within the A-V junction.

junction. This is reflected by an even shallower slope when compared with Diagram A.

Diagram C of Fig. 135 represents A-V block—an interruption of conduction within the A-V node.

Note that Diagrams A, B and C together would represent sinus rhythm complicated by 3:2 second degree A-V block of the Wenckebach Type (see Chapter 18).

Diagram D of Fig. 135 represents phasic aberrant ventricular conduction—the abnormal intermittent intraventricular conduction of a supraventricular impulse.

Diagram E of Fig. 135 represents a ventricular impulse with retrograde A-V conduction to the atria.

Diagram F of Fig. 135 represents a ventricular impulse which is dissociated from a near-synchronous sinus impulse. Interference with consequent A-V dissociation occurs within the A-V node.

SECTION 2
DISORDERS OF
IMPULSE FORMATION

Sinus Rhythms
Ectopic Atrial Rhythms
A-V Nodal Rhythms
Ventricular Rhythms
Parasystole

Chapter 12
Sinus Rhythms

SINUS ARRHYTHMIA · SINUS TACHYCARDIA ·
SINUS BRADYCARDIA

SINUS ARRHYTHMIA

Sinus arrhythmia is characterized by alternating periods of slow and rapid rates; it is due to an irregular fluctuating discharge of the S-A node. The condition is most commonly associated with the phases of respiration—**respiratory sinus arrhythmia.** The periods of faster rate occur towards the end of inspiration, and the periods of slower rate towards the end of expiration, The mechanism is mediated by reflex stimulation of the vagus nerve from receptors in the lungs.

Diagnosis. The impulses arise from the S-A node and the P waves are therefore normal; the subsequent course of the sinus impulse, in the absence of a conduction disturbance, is also normal, resulting in a normal P–R interval and QRST complex. The arrhythmia is thus characterized by **normal P-QRST complexes** with alternating periods of gradually lengthening and gradually shortening P–P intervals (Fig. 136).

Sinus arrhythmia is accentuated by vagotonic procedures, such as digitalis administration and carotid sinus compression. It is abolished by vagolytic procedures, viz. exercise, atropine and amyl nitrite.

SIGNIFICANCE

Respiratory sinus arrhythmia is a normal physiological pheno-

154

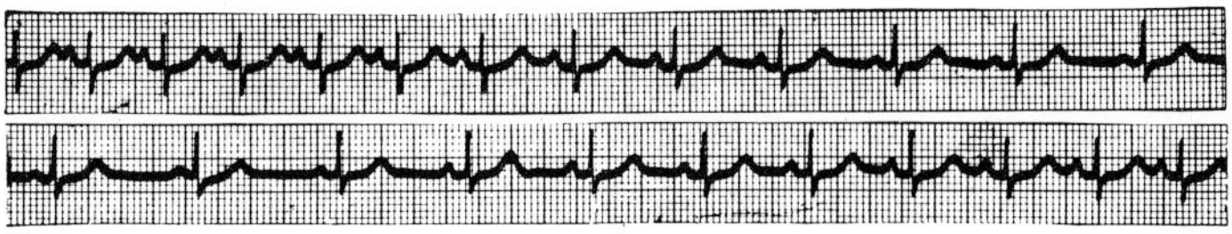

Fig. 136. Electrocardiogram (continuous recording of Standard lead II) showing sinus arrhythmia.

menon, and is most marked in young persons. It may cause considerable irregularity of the pulse in childhood.

SINUS TACHYCARDIA

Sinus tachycardia occurs when the S-A node discharges at a rate faster than 100 per minute in the adult. The normal 'resting' rate in infants averages 120–130 beats per minute, slowing gradually to reach the adult rate at puberty.

Diagnosis. Sinus tachycardia is, in the absence of a complicating conduction disturbance, characterized by **normal P-QRST complexes which are recorded in rapid succession.** It varies with emotion, respiration and exercise. Vagotonic procedures, e.g. carotid sinus compression, results in slight but gradual slowing.

SIGNIFICANCE

Sinus tachycardia is the normal physiological response to exercise and emotion. A sinus tachycardia that persists at rest is usually an expression of some underlying disorder. It occurs in anxiety states, thyrotoxicosis, toxaemia, cardiac failure (as a result of an increased Bainbridge reflex) and in acute carditis. It is a normal accompaniment of fever. The sinus rate will increase by 8 beats per minute for every one degree increase in temperature (Holzmann, 1965). A diminution in oxygen saturation, as occurs at high altitudes or in association with congenital heart disease, will also cause a sinus tachycardia. Failure to develop sinus tachycardia with exercise or fever may be an expression of structural nodal disease—the so-called sick sinus syndrome (see Chapter 26). It may be caused by the administration of adrenaline, atropine, caffeine and amyl nitrate.

SINUS BRADYCARDIA

Sinus bradycardia occurs when the S-A node discharges at a rate slower than 60 per minute.

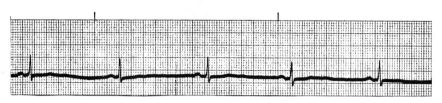

Fig. 137. Electrocardiogram (Standard lead I) showing marked sinus bradycardia. *Note*: there are just over two cardiac cycles, or R–R intervals, in every 3 sec—fifteen large squares (every fifteenth large square is marked by a vertical line on the upper border of the graph paper); the rate is, therefore, just over 40 per minute.

Diagnosis. Sinus bradycardia, in the absence of a complicating conduction disturbance, characterized by **normal P-QRST complexes which are recorded in slow succession** (Figs. 132 and 137). It is commonly associated with respiratory sinus arrhythmia.

SIGNIFICANCE

Sinus bradycardia occurs as a normal phenomenon in athletes. Slowing of the sinus rate—at times to bradycardic levels—is the physiological response to sleep. Sinus bradycardia is accentuated by digitalis and vagotonic procedures, such as carotid sinus compression. The rate quickens gradually with exercise, emotion and amyl nitrite.

Sinus bradycardia is associated with myxoedema, obstructive jaundice (the effect of direct action of the bile salts on the S-A node), uraemia, increased intracranial pressure, and glaucoma (increased and persistent oculocardiac reflex).

A common present-day cause of sinus bradycardia is the administration of beta-blocking agents.

When the aforementioned causes of sinus bradycardia can be excluded, the presence of structural disease of the S-A node should be considered. This is one of the manifestations of Structural Nodal Disease or the so-called Sick Sinus Syndrome (see Chapter 26).

See also the differential diagnosis of a slow regular ventricular rhythm (page 296).

Chapter 13
Ectopic Atrial Rhythms
ATRIAL EXTRASYSTOLES · PAROXYSMAL ATRIAL TACHYCARDIA ·
ATRIAL FIBRILLATION · ATRIAL FLUTTER · ATRIAL ESCAPE

ATRIAL EXTRASYSTOLES

An atrial extrasystole is due to the **premature** discharge of an **ectopic atrial focus.** It has the following characteristics:

1. THE P WAVE IS BIZARRE

The discharge arises from an ectopic atrial focus, i.e. from a point other than the S-A node. The activation front thus travels across the atria by unusual pathways resulting in an abnormal or bizarre P′ wave—a P′ wave that is different from the sinus P wave and which may be *pointed, notched, diphasic* or *inverted* (Figs. 138, 139, 140, 141 and 219).

2. THE BIZARRE P′ WAVE IS PREMATURE

The ectopic impulse arises in the diastolic period of the preceding sinus beat and is thus recorded earlier than the next anticipated sinus P wave.

3. THE COMPENSATORY PAUSE IS INCOMPLETE (see Fig. 138)

(*a*) The ectopic impulse reaches and discharges the sinus node prematurely—position A in Fig. 138.

(*b*) The recharge of the S-A node thus begins at position A and the next sinus discharge occurs at position C. (Had the sinus node not been prematurely discharged, the recharge would begin at position B and the following discharge would then occur at position D.)

(*c*) The next normal sinus impulse, therefore, does not occur as scheduled, viz. at position B; for the S-A node must pass through a *complete recovery cycle* before it can discharge again. This recovery cycle is sometimes termed the return cycle.

(*d*) The basic rhythm of the S-A node is thus disturbed and a pause follows the ectopic beat—the compensatory pause. This pause,

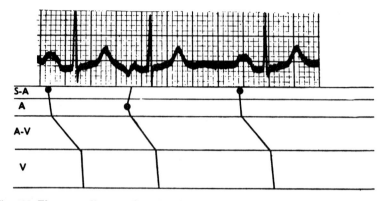

Fig. 138. Electrocardiogram (Standard lead II) showing sinus rhythm complicated by an atrial extrasystole as reflected by the bizarre premature P′ wave; There is first degree A-V block of the sinus impulse as reflected by a prolonged P–R interval or 0.24 sec (six small squares); The sinus P wave is widened and plateau-shaped reflecting left atrial enlargement—a P mitrale. From a case of mitral stenosis on digitalis therapy. The large black dots indicate impulse origin. S-A = sino-atrial level; A = atrial level; A-V = A-V nodal level; V = ventricular level.

however, is incomplete, i.e. it does not fully compensate for the prematurity of the extrasystole. This means that the sum of the pre- and post-ectopic intervals (Y–Z in Figs. 138 and 139) is *less than* the sum of two consecutive normal intervals (X–Y in Figs. 138 and 139).

Compare those events with those occasioned by a ventricular extrasystole where the sinus rhythm is not disturbed and where the compensatory pause is consequently complete (Fig. 158).

It must, nevertheless, be stressed that the aforementioned theoretical appraisal of the compensatory mechanism does not often apply.

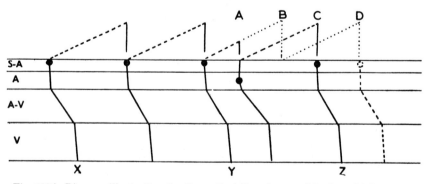

Fig. 139A. Diagram illustrating the theoretical disturbance of rhythm which occurs with an atrial extrasystole. The dotted lines indicate the recharge of the S-A node. The large black dots indicate impulse origin (see text).

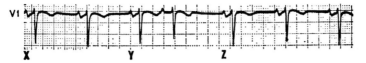

Fig. 139B. Electrocardiogram (lead V1) showing normal sinus rhythm complicated by an atrial extrasystole. This is reflected by the fourth P wave which is premature and bizarre: pointed, narrow and entirely positive. The compensatory pause is incomplete, i.e. the sum of the pre- and post-ectopic intervals (interval Y–Z) is *less than* the sum of two consecutive sinus intervals (interval X–Y).

This is because of the phenomenon of pacemaker depression as a result of its premature discharge. The premature discharge of any pacemaker will tend to depress it momentarily. In the case of an atrial extrasystole, the extrasystolic impulse discharges the sinus pacemaker prematurely and thus tends to depress it momentarily. The return sinus cycle which constitutes the compensatory pause may consequently be longer than normal. This principle may be used to assess the function of the S-A node in structural nodal disease or the so-called Sick Sinus Syndrome (see Chapter 26). If the return cycle is longer than 25 per cent of the original basic cycle, structural S-A nodal disease is probably present.

4. CONDUCTION OF THE ATRIAL EXTRASYSTOLIC IMPULSE

(a) A-V conduction

Conduction of the atrial impulse to the ventricles depends upon the recovery state of the A-V node when the impulse reaches it. Thus:

(i) The atrial impulse may be conducted with:

(a) A *normal P–R interval* (Fig. 140).

(b) A *prolonged P–R interval.* This will occur if the prematurity of the extrasystole is such that it encounters a partially refractory A-V node and is thus delayed.

(c) A *relatively short P–R interval,* i.e. a P–R interval that is

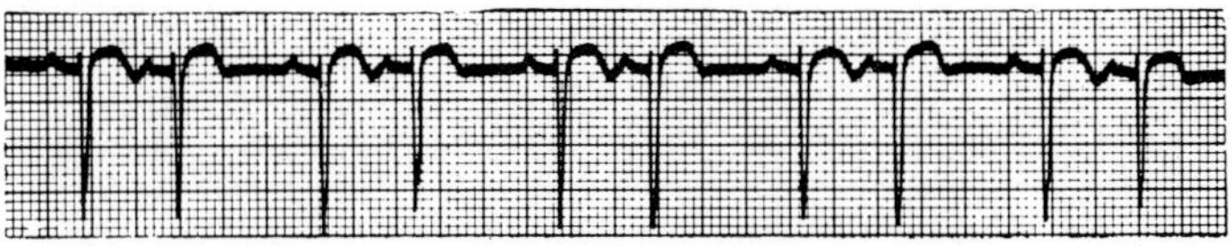

Fig. 140. Electrocardiogram showing alternate conducted atrial extrasystoles causing both atrial and ventricular bigeminal rhythm.

slightly shorter than that of the conducted sinus beat (Fig. 138). This will occur when the extrasystole arises from a focus that is relatively low or distal in the atria and thus reaches the A-V node quickly.

(ii) The ectopic impulse may be *blocked*: A very early impulse may find the A-V node refractory and conduction to the ventricles is therefore blocked. A blocked or non-conducted atrial extrasystole is characterized by an abnormal and premature P wave that is *not* followed by a QRS complex (Figs. 63, 141, 207, 219). The abnormal P wave may not be obvious, especially if it is superimposed on the T wave of the preceding sinus beat; as a result, the T wave is slightly deformed—a little more pointed or slightly notched (Fig. 219, top strip). And if this premature abnormal P wave is not observed, the pause may be mistakenly diagnosed as due to S-A block. Thus, in all cases where a long pause is apparently due to S-A block, the preceding T wave must be compared with other T waves and critically examined for even the slightest deformity.

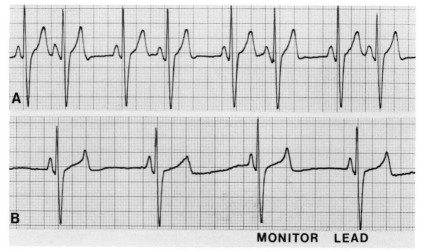

MONITOR LEAD

Fig. 141. (A) Electrocardiogram (Monitor lead) showing sinus rhythm complicated by alternate atrial extrasystoles. These are reflected by the premature P′ waves which are slightly different in configuation from the sinus P waves. These atrial extrasystoles are conducted to the ventricles. This results in a ventricular bigeminal rhythm.
(B) Electrocardiogram recorded from the same patient showing sinus rhythm complicated by very premature atrial extrasystoles. The P′ waves of these atrial extrasystoles are superimposed upon, and distort, the T waves. The atrial extrasystoles are not conducted due to their marked prematurity. This results in slow regular ventricular rhythm.

(*b*) *Intraventricular conduction*

After passing through the A-V node, intraventricular conduction of the ectopic impulse may take one of the following forms:

(i) *Normal intraventricular conduction*: the impulse is conducted through both bundle branches and results in a normal QRS complex (Figs. 138, 140, 141 and 142).

(ii) *Aberrant ventricular conduction*: the impulse reaches the bundle branches when only one has fully recovered. The impulse is then conducted through one bundle branch only resulting in a bundle branch block pattern. This may be associated with a hemiblock (Figs. 219 and 221, and see Chapter 18 on Phasic Aberrant Ventricular Conduction).

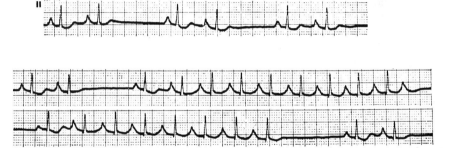

Fig. 142. *Top strip*: Electrocardiogram (Standard lead II) showing sinus rhythm complicated by alternate conducted atrial extrasystoles resulting in both atrial and ventricular bigeminal rhythm.

    Bottom two strips: (continuous recording; a later section of the same electrocardiogram) showing sinus rhythm with atrial extrasystoles (beginning and end of the record), and two paroxysms of extrasystolic atrial tachycardia arising from the same ectopic atrial focus as the atrial extrasystoles.

SIGNIFICANCE OF ATRIAL EXTRASYSTOLES

Atrial extrasystoles may be found in association with *chronic rheumatic valvular disease*—mitral stenosis and mitral incompetence; in coronary artery disease, in hyperthyroidism and in digitalis intoxication. Atrial extrasystoles may appear occasionally with viral infections. Occasional atrial extrasystoles may occur in normal individuals.

Alternate conducted atrial extrasystoles are a cause of both atrial and ventricular bigeminal rhythm (Fig. 140). Frequent multifocal atrial extrasystoles often herald atrial fibrillation. Three or more consecutive atrial extrasystoles constitute a paroxysmal atrial tachycardia.

SUMMARY

Timing   premature
                                                compensatory pause
                                                theoretically incomplete

Atrial conduction   abnormal—bizarre P wave

A-V conduction   blocked   conducted

                                                        P–R interval

                              normal   prolonged   short

Intraventricular conduction   normal   aberrant

EXTRASYSTOLIC—PAROXYSMAL—ATRIAL TACHYCARDIA

Paroxysmal atrial tachycardia is due to the rapid discharge of an ectopic atrial focus: a series of three or more rapidly occurring, regular and consecutive atrial extrasystoles.

MECHANISM AND ELECTROCARDIOGRAPHIC CHARACTERISTICS

1. ATRIAL ACTIVATION

The atrial focus is ectopic and the course of atrial depolarization is, therefore, abnormal. This results in an *abnormally shaped* P wave (Figs. 142 and 143).

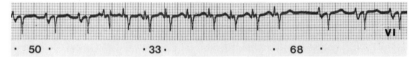

Fig. 143. Electrocardiogram (lead V1) showing the following features: (*a*) Sinus tachycardia as reflected by the first 2 and last 3 beats of the tracing. The P–P intervals measure 0.50 sec representing a rate of 120 per minute. (*b*) Left atrial enlargement as reflected by the marked delayed terminal negativity of the sinus beats. (*c*) Extrasystolic atrial tachycardia as reflected by the fourth to twelfth beats of the tracing. The P′ waves are bizarre: narrow and sharply pointed, reflecting an ectopic atrial origin. The P′–P′ intervals measure 0.33 sec representing a rate of 182 per minute. Intraventricular conduction is the same as that associated with the sinus beats. The post tachycardia pause measures 0.68 sec. This is more than a 25% increase of the basic sinus cycle of 0.50 sec and thus reflects possible structural disease of the S-A node.

2. A-V CONDUCTION

On reaching the A-V node, the atrial impulse may be conducted as follows:

(*a*) With *normal A-V conduction* resulting in a normal P–R interval.

(*b*) With a shorter than normal P–R interval (Fig. 143).

(*c*) With *first degree A-V block*. Because of the rapid ectopic discharge rate and conduction frequency through the A-V node there may be insufficient time for complete recovery of the A-V node. The

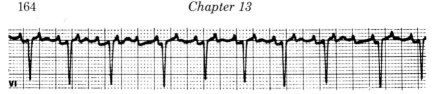

Fig. 144. Electrocardiogram (lead V1) showing extrasystolic atrial tachycardia with varying second degree A-V block: 'P.A.T. with block'. The P′ waves are bizarre. The P′–P′ interval measures 0.24 sec, representing an atrial rate of 250 per minute. The A-V conduction ratios vary between 3:1 and 2:1.

atrial impulse is thus conducted with delay as reflected by first degree A-V block (Fig. 142).

(*d*) With *second degree A-V block*. The extrasystolic tachycardia may be so rapid that its cycle is shorter than the A-V nodal refractory period. When this occurs, every second atrial impulse is blocked resulting in a 2:1 A-V block. The atrial tachycardia may also be associated with more complex forms of second degree A-V block, e.g. (*a*) a 3:2 block, possibly of the Wenckebach type or (*b*) a fluctuating ratio in the degree of A-V block, e.g. 3:2, 2:1, 2:1, 3:2, etc. (Fig. 144). This form is frequently due to digitalis intoxication. This is known as paroxysmal tachycardia with block, and is sometimes abbreviated to the cryptic term of 'P.A.T. with block'.

3. INTRAVENTRICULAR CONDUCTION

On reaching the ventricles, the atrial impulses may be conducted as follows:

(*a*) With *normal intraventricular conduction*. Intraventricular conduction may be normal. This will manifest with a series of normal QRS complexes which are inscribed in rapid and regular succession, each related to a preceding ectopic atrial P wave (Figs. 142, 143 and 144).

(*b*) With *phasic aberrant ventricular conduction*. The impulses of the atrial tachycardia may be conducted with phasic aberrant ventricular conduction (see Chapter 25). The atrial impulses are conducted through one bundle branch only, resulting in the bizarre QRS complex of right or left bundle branch block with possible associated hemiblock (see Chapter 25). The succession of bizarre QRS complexes may mimic ectopic ventricular tachycardia (Figs. 224 and 227).

4. THE EFFECT ON THE S-T SEGMENT AND T WAVE

Any tachycardia may result in relative coronary insufficiency which will, of course, be worse if the coronary arteries are diseased. The coronary insufficiency manifests as S-T segment depression and T wave inversion in those leads where the QRS complexes are dominantly upright. These changes are present during the tachycardia and may persist for hours or days *after the tachycardia has ceased*—the **post-tachycardia syndrome.**

SUPRAVENTRICULAR TACHYCARDIA

At times, a tachycardia presents with narrow, normal or relatively normal QRS complexes, thereby suggesting a supraventricular origin, but identification of the P′ waves is difficult, or the P′ to QRS relationship cannot be established with certainty. The rhythm may then be conveniently referred to as **supraventricular tachycardia.** Most of these cases are almost certainly reciprocating tachycardia, especially so since, under this circumstance, there is a 1:1 relationship (see Chapter 20).

EXTRASYSTOLIC ATRIAL TACHYCARDIA

SUMMARY

Atrial conduction: Abnormal P′ waves *preceding* the QRS complexes

A-V conduction:	first degree A-V block	second degree A-V block	normal conduction (uncommon)

Intraventricular conduction:	normal	aberrant

S-T segment: frequently depressed

T wave: frequently inverted

ATRIAL FIBRILLATION

Under normal circumstances the sinus impulse is transmitted uniformly, evenly and contiguously to all parts of the atria. In atrial fibrillation *excitation and recovery of the atria are disorganized and chaotic*. The atria are functionally fractionated into a chaotic state of numerous tissue islets in various stages of excitation and recovery. These numerous excitatory wavelets or stimuli course irregularly through atria and reach the A-V node at frequent and irregular intervals; the rate of such impulses which reach the A-V node may range from 400 to 600 per minute. The A-V node can only conduct some of these stimuli, because, following conduction of one such stimulus, it is refractory for a short period, and impulses reaching the A-V node during this period are blocked. As the refractory period of the A-V node varies with such factors as vagal stimulation, res-piration, emotion, exercise, and incomplete or partial penetration of the atrial impulses into the A-V node (concealed conduction), transmission to the ventricles is irregular. All cases of atrial fibrillation are thus associated with some form of second degree A-V block.

Intraventricular conduction of the impulses from the fibrillating atria may, at times, be associated with phasic aberrant ventricular conduction (see Chapter 25).

In untreated cases the ventricular response, i.e. the ventricular rate is usually about 120–150 per minute. Digitalis slows, i.e. diminishes the ventricular response by *increasing the refractory period of the A-V node.*

The initiation of atrial fibrillation is the result of *very early stimulation* of the atria, and is usually due to a very premature atrial extrasystole (Fig. 146). Maintenance of the fibrillation is favoured by a *large mass of atrial tissue* as is commonly found in association with cardiac failure.

ELECTROCARDIOGRAPHIC MANIFESTATIONS

The atrial deflections are irregular and chaotic resulting in a *ragged baseline* with numerous rounded or spiked waves of varying shape, height and width (Fig. 145).

In long-standing cases of atrial fibrillation the deflections may be of low amplitude and the baseline may be almost straight with minimal smooth low-amplitude undulations (Fig. 145A).

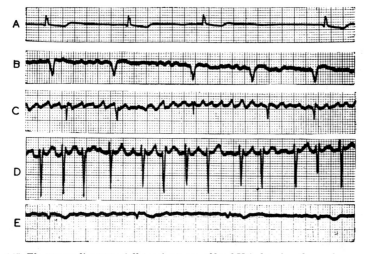

Fig. 145. Electrocardiograms (all tracings are of lead V1) showing the various manifestations of atrial fibrillation (A) shows long-standing atrial fibrillation. Note (*a*) the smooth, slightly undulating baseline; (*b*) the slow and irregular ventricular response; (*c*) the digitalis effect in the S-T segment. (B) and (C) are examples of a coarser, more recent fibrillation with a relatively slow ventricular response. Note the irregular and ragged baseline. (D) shows the same features as (C) but with a rapid ventricular response. (E) shows atrial fibrillation with complete A-V block. Note the *regularly* spaced QRS complexes.

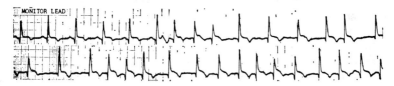

Fig. 146. Electrocardiogram (Monitor lead) showing: 1. Sinus rhythm. This is represented by the first six beats. 2. An atrial extrasystole. This occurs immediately after, and deforms the S-T segment of, the sixth beat. 3. Atrial fibrillation. The atrial extrasystole occurs very prematurely, i.e. during the vulnerable phase of the atria, and thus precipitates atrial fibrillation—the rest of the tracing. Note the chaotic baseline due to deformity by the *f* waves of the atrial fibrillation, and the irregular ventricular response.

SIGNIFICANCE

Atrial fibrillation occurs in mitral and tricuspid valvular disease, in coronary artery disease, hyperthyroidism and in approximately 30 per cent of cases of constrictive pericarditis.

Paroxysmal atrial fibrillation occurs in the W-P-W syndrome (Chapter 21) and hyperthyroidism.

Atrial fibrillation may occur in the absence of any other manifestation or organic heart disease and has been termed 'Lone Auricular Fibrillation' (Evans & Swann, 1954[1]). It usually occurs in young individuals who have no evidence of coronary artery disease. A familial incidence has also been reported. The phenomenon is probably due to the presence of an anomalous or additional A-V nodal by-pass congenital in origin—which permits rapid (reciprocal) return of the sinus impulse to the atria (Schamroth & Krikler, 1967[2]); a mechanism analogous to the Wolff-Parkinson-White syndrome (see Chapter 21). The rapidly returning impulse constitutes a source of very premature stimulation, and may precipitate atrial fibrillation.

ATRIAL FLUTTER

Atrial flutter is the expression of a *rapid* and *regular* atrial excitation. This excitation may be due to two mechanisms either of which may be operative, viz.

1.   *A circus movement* that results from a continuous, self-perpetuating circular path of excitation coursing around the orifices of the superior and inferior vena cavae. This is the most likely mechanism.

2.   *A focal discharge*—the rapid discharge of an ectopic atrial focus; similar to that of extrasystolic—paroxysmal—atrial tachycardia.

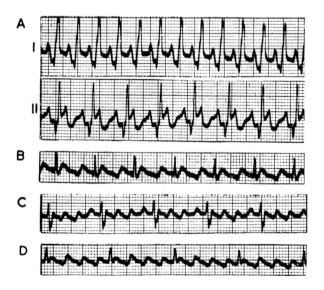

Fig. 147. Electrocardiograms (all tracings of Standard lead II) showing the various forms of flutter. (A) I shows atrial flutter with a 1:1 A-V response. (A) II is from the same patient after treatment with digitalis and shows a 2:1 A-V response. (B) shows atrial flutter with a 2:1 A-V response. (C) and (D) show atrial flutter with a 4:1 A-V response. Note (*a*) the rapid atrial rate; (*b*) the wide 'saw-tooth' deflections; (*c*) the absent or barely noticeable baseline.

The ventricular response to this rapid atrial activity depends upon the efficacy of A-V conduction. Occasionally, every atrial impulse or excitatory circuit is conducted to the ventricles—a 1:1 response—resulting in a very fast ventricular rate (Fig. 147A). More commonly, second degree A-V block is present, e.g. in a ratio of 2:1, 4:1, 6:1 or 8:1, resulting in a relatively slow ventricular rate (Fig. 147—A II, B, C and D). Even ratios—2:1, 4:1 or 6:1—are commoner than odd ratios—3:1 or 5:1. Sometimes the conduction ratio fluctuates, e.g. from 4:1 to 6:1 to 2:1 ratios, etc.; this results in completely irregular ventricular rhythm. Regular 3:2 conduction ratios will result in ventricular bigeminal rhythm. Alternating 4:1 and 2:1 conduction ratios will also result in bigeminal rhythm (Fig. 237). Atrial flutter may also be complicated by complete A-V block.

Intraventricular conduction of the flutter impulses may at times be associated with phasic aberrant ventricular conduction (see Chapter 18 and Fig. 237).

ELECTROCARDIOGRAPHIC CHARACTERISTICS

The cardinal sign of atrial flutter is the presence of regular, undulating closely spaced but relatively wide atrial deflections or flutter—'F'—waves affecting the whole baseline and resulting in a *regular, corrugated or saw-tooth appearance* (Figs. 147 and 237). The isoelectric level between flutter waves is much shortened and is frequently not discernible. This manifestation is usually best seen in the frontal plane leads, especially Standard leads II and III, and lead AVF. The F waves are usually negative in these leads, thereby reflecting a superior F wave axis and caudo-cranial atrial activation. Lead V1, in contrast to the frontal plane leads, usually shows an iso-electric shelf. The F waves also tend to be narrow. The T waves are usually masked or deformed by the flutter waves.

Flutter waves are best seen in Standard lead II and lead V1.

The QRS complexes are normal unless there is coincidental bundle branch block, or a complicating phasic aberrant ventricular conduction (see Chapter 25 and Figs. 237 and 238).

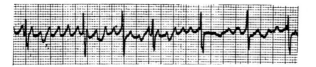

Fig. 148. Electrocardiogram illustrating so-called *flutter-fibrillation*.

When the saw-tooth appearance shows some irregularity or distortion suggestive of atrial fibrillation, the condition is sometimes referred to as *impure-flutter* or *flutter-fibrillation* (Fig. 148). It is doubtful, however, whether this represents a separate or finite entity; examples of this so-called condition are probably cases of uncomplicated atrial fibrillation.

Digitalis often converts atrial flutter to atrial fibrillation due to a shortening of the atrial refractory period. This may be followed by conversion to normal rhythm when the digitalis is stopped.

SIGNIFICANCE

Atrial flutter is commonly associated with chronic rheumatic valvular disease and ischaemic, hypertensive and pulmonary heart disease. Like paroxysmal atrial tachycardia, it has an abrupt onset and termination. Succeeding attacks of atrial flutter tend to last longer, however, and frequently precede permanent atrial fibrillation. Atrial flutter is more responsive to electrical cardioversion than any other tachyarrhythmia.

ATRIAL ESCAPE

This is discussed in Chapter 22.

REFERENCES

1 Evans W. & Swann P. (1954) Lone auricular fibrillation. *Brit. Heart J.* **16,** 189.
2 Schamroth L. & Krikler D. M. (1967) The problem of lone atrial fibrillation. *S.A. Med. J.* **41,** 502.

Chapter 14
A-V Nodal Rhythms

A-V NODAL EXTRASYSTOLES · EXTRASYSTOLIC—
PAROXYSMAL—A-V NODAL TACHYCARDIA ·
IDIONODAL TACHYCARDIA · A-V NODAL ESCAPE

THE CONDUCTION SEQUENCES OF
A-V NODAL RHYTHMS

An impulse arising within the A-V node or junction may have the following conduction sequences:
1. The nodal impulse may be conducted to the atria and ventricles (Fig. 149A, B and C).
2. The A-V nodal impulse may be conducted to the ventricles only, retrograde conduction to the atria being blocked or impeded by interference from a near-synchronous sinus impulse (Fig. 149D).
3. Occasionally, anterograde conduction of the A-V nodal impulse to the ventricles may be blocked or impeded by interference.

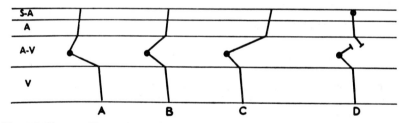

Fig. 149. Diagram illustrating various conduction mechanisms in A-V nodal rhythm (A) illustrates an A-V nodal beat with earlier retrograde conduction. (B) illustrates an A-V nodal beat with equal anterograde and retrograde conduction times. (C) illustrates an A-V nodal beat with late retrograde conduction. (D) illustrates an A-V nodal beat complicated by interference, resulting in a dissociated beat. The large black dots indicate impulse origin. S-A = sino-atrial level; A = atrial level; A-V = A-V nodal level; V = ventricular level.

1. A-V NODAL RHYTHM WITH CONDUCTION TO ATRIA AND VENTRICLES

The QRS and P' wave forms

When the A-V nodal impulse is conducted to the atria and ventricles concomitantly, conduction to the ventricles usually proceeds along

171

normal A-V conduction pathways resulting in a normal or near-normal QRST complex. Conduction to the atria, however, occurs retrogradely, i.e. the direction of atrial depolarization is reversed, and occurs from below upwards. As a result, *the P′ wave is inverted in leads where it is normally upright* and vice versa, i.e. it is inverted in Standard leads II and III, and lead AVF, upright in leads AVR and AVL, and usually equiphasic in Standard lead I (Fig. 152). In other words, the P′ wave vector is directed superiorly to the region of − 80° to − 90° on the frontal plane hexaxial reference system. This 'retrograde' P′ wave is usually sharply pointed, narrow and dominantly positive in lead V1. This contrasts with the normal diphasic sinus P wave.

RELATIONSHIP OF P WAVE TO QRS COMPLEX

Depending upon the relative velocity of anterograde and retrograde conduction, the P wave may *precede, follow, or occur synchronously with, and thus be hidden within, the QRS complex.*

(*a*) If retrograde conduction to the atria is relatively faster than anterograde conduction to the ventricles, the 'retrograde' P′ wave will *precede* the QRS complex; the P′–R interval is shortened (Figs. 149A and 150).

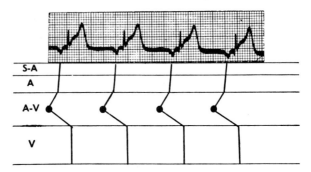

Fig. 150. Electrocardiogram (Standard lead II) showing A-V nodal rhythm with earlier retrograde conduction. An inverted P wave precedes each QRS complex. Large black dots indicate impulse origin.

(*b*) If anterograde conduction to the ventricles is relatively faster than retrograde conduction to the atria the 'retrograde' P′ wave will *follow* the QRS complex (Figs. 149C, 151 and 152).

(*c*) If conduction to the atria and ventricles occurs at the same rate the 'retrograde' P′ wave will be recorded at the same time as, and be *hidden within*, the QRS complex (Fig. 149B).

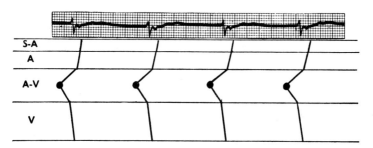

Fig. 151. Electrocardiogram (Standard lead II) showing A-V nodal rhythm with late retrograde conduction. *Note*: an inverted P wave follows each QRS complex. Large black dots indicate impulse origin.

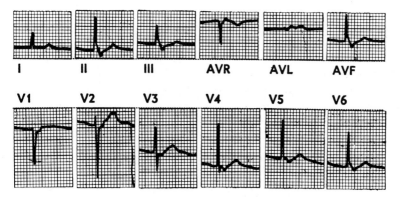

Fig. 152. Electrocardiogram showing A-V nodal rhythm with late retrograde conduction to, and activation of, the atria. Note (*a*) the P waves follow each QRS complex; (*b*) the P waves are inverted in Standard leads II and lead AVF.

2. A-V NODAL RHYTHM WITH CONDUCTION TO THE
VENTRICLES ONLY

In this condition, conduction to the ventricles proceeds along normal pathways resulting in a normal QRST complex. Retrograde conduction to the atria, however, does not occur, because of—

(*a*) a true retrograde block of the A-V nodal impulse (Fig. 215) or

(*b*) interference with retrograde conduction of the A-V nodal impulse by a concomitant sinus impulse (Figs. 153, 155, 156, 207, 208 and 209).

In both these conditions, the sinus P waves are dissociated from the AV nodal QRS complexes.

These manifestations of A-V nodal rhythm thus constitute a form of A-V dissociation (see section on A-V dissociation, Chapter 23).

THE FORMS OF A-V NODAL RHYTHM

An A-V nodal or junctional rhythm may take the form of:
1. An **A-V nodal extrasystole** (Fig. 153).
2. An **A-V nodal escape beat** (Figs. 207 and 209).
3. **Extrasystolic—paroxysmal—A-V nodal tachycardia** (Fig. 155).
4. **Idionodal tachycardia** (Fig. 156).

Note. The P-QRS relationship in all these A-V nodal rhythms may take any of the forms described above, viz. a 'retrograde' P wave is related to and may precede, follow, or be hidden within, the QRS complex; or a sinus P wave is unrelated to or dissociated from, the QRS complex.

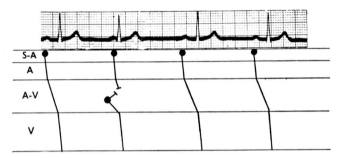

Fig. 153. Electrocardiogram showing an A-V nodal extrasystole. The first, third and fourth QRS complexes result from normal sinus beats conducted with first degree A-V block (P–R interval = 0.24 sec). The second QRS complex occurs prematurely and has virtually the same shape as the other QRS complexes; it is dissociated from the second sinus P wave. Black dots indicate impulse origin; S-A = sino-atrial level; A atrial level; A-V = A-V nodal level; V = ventricular level.

1. A-V NODAL EXTRASYSTOLES

An A-V nodal extrasystole is the expression of an impulse which arises prematurely in the A-V node. If the A-V nodal extrasystole occurs with retrograde spread to the atria, the sinus node is usually discharged prematurely and the compensatory pause is, theoretically, incomplete. The sequence of events is similar to that occurring with an atrial extrasystole (see page 157).

If the A-V nodal extrasystole occurs without retrograde acti-

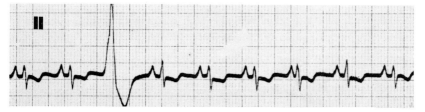

Fig. 154. The electrocardiogram (Standard lead II) shows: 1. Sinus tachycardia. The P–P intervals measure 0.58 sec to 0.60 sec, representing a rate of 100 to 104 beats per minute. 2. A ventricular extasystole. This is reflected by the bizarre, abnormal and premature QRS complex which is unrelated to the P waves. The coupling interval measures 0.43 sec. 3. An A-V nodal extrasystole. This is reflected by the seventh QRS complex (the sixth normal QRS complex). This QRS complex is normal—reflecting a supraventricular origin—and premature; the coupling interval (R–R interval) measures 0.53 sec. The QRS complex is unrelated to the preceding P wave. Note the shortening of the P to R′ interval. This A-V nodal extrasystole is thus dissociated from the concomitant sinus P wave, the two impulses meet within the A-V node and interfere with each other's mutual progress. This is an example of a so-called 'Main-stem' extrasystole.

vation of the atria (Fig. 153), there is no interference with the sinus discharge, and the compensatory pause is complete (Fig. 154). The sequence of events is similar to that occurring with most forms of ventricular extrasystoles (see page 183). A-V nodal extrasystoles have the same significance as atrial extrasystoles (see page 161).

2. A-V NODAL ESCAPE BEAT

(This is discussed in Chapter 22.)

3. EXTRASYSTOLIC—PAROXYSMAL—A-V NODAL TACHYCARDIA

This may be defined as a succession of three or more A-V nodal extrasystoles (Fig. 155). and has the same significance as a paroxysmal atrial tachycardia.

Unlike idionodal tachycardia (see below), extrasystolic A-V nodal tachycardia has an abrupt onset and termination. Extrasystolic tachycardia is relatively uncommon.

4. IDIONODAL TACHYCARDIA

(Synonym: Non-paroxysmal A-V Nodal Tachycardia)

Idionodal tachycardia is the expression of an accelerated inherent

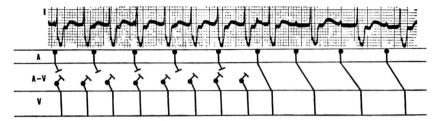

Fig. 155. Electrocardiogram (Standard lead I) showing: 1. Extrasystolic—paroxysmal—A-V nodal tachycardia, represented by the first eight QRS complexes. 2. A-V dissociation: the QRS complexes bear no relationship to the concomitant sinus rhythm; the P waves may be seen just before the QRS complexes or superimposed upon the S-T segments. 3. A ventricular capture beat. The 9th QRS complex is premature and is related to the preceding P wave. This represents the conduction to, and capture of, the ventricles by the preceding sinus impulse. 4. Sinus rhythm with first degree A-V block. The capture beat terminates the tachycardia, and sinus rhythm ensues. The P–R interval measures 0.22 sec. *Note:* (*a*) The QRS complexes of the conducted sinus impulses are identical to the QRS complexes of the ectopic tachycardia. This establishes the A-V nodal origin of the tachycardia, since the impulses of the tachycardia must have followed the same intraventricular pathway as that used by the sinus impulses. (*b*) The sudden termination of the ectopic tachycardia reflects its extrasystolic character.

idionodal rhythm, an enhancement of the inherent automaticity of a latent potential idionodal pacemaker—analogous to the enhancement of an idioventricular pacemaker in idioventricular tachycardia. The principles governing these arrhythmias are discussed in the section on idioventricular tachycardia (see page 191). The rhythm was first described by Pick & Dominguez (1957)[1] who termed it 'non-paroxysmal A-V nodal tachycardia' to distinguish it from the extrasystolic or paroxysmal forms of A-V nodal tachycardia.

Electrocardiographic manifestations

The diagnosis of idionodal tachycardia is based on the following criteria:

1. CRITERIA FOR THE ESTABLISHMENT OF A-V NODAL ORIGIN

This is based upon:

A. The presence of a normal QRS complex or a QRS complex that has the same configuration as that of the conducted sinus impulse.

B. The conduction sequences characteristically associated with A-V nodal rhythms (see page 171).

2. AN ENHANCED IDIONODAL RATE

The normal inherent idionodal rate is usually in the range of 50 to 60 beats per minute. Allowing for some measure of overlap, an idionodal tachycardia may be arbitrarily defined as an idionodal rhythm whose rate exceeds 70 beats per minute. The rate of an idionodal tachycardia is most commonly between 70 and 100 beats per minute.

3. A PROPENSITY TO A-V DISSOCIATION

As the enhanced idionodal rhythm is usually in the same rate-range as that of the sinus rhythm, concomitant discharge is frequent, and A-V dissociation is, therefore, a common occurrence (Figs. 156 and 215).

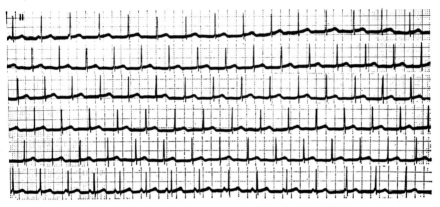

Fig. 156. The electrocardiogram (a continuous strip of Standard lead II) shows: 1. *Sinus rhythm.* This is evident at the beginning of the top strip and in the bottom strip where the P wave can be identified. The P–P intervals range from 0.60 sec to 0.70 sec reflecting a rate of 86 to 100 beats per minute—an expression of minimal sinus arrhythmia. 2. *Idionodal tachycardia.* This is reflected by the QRS complexes which are normal and bear no relationship to the P waves. The R–R intervals measure 0.64 sec, representing a rate of 94 beats per minute. 3. *A-V dissociation.* The P waves and the QRS complexes are dissociated or unrelated. At the beginning of the recording, the P waves are seen to 'move into' the QRS complexes, i.e. the sinus rhythm attains the same rate as the idionodal rhythm. The two rhythms maintain this rate for about 45 seconds during which the P waves are hidden within the QRS complexes. The two rhythms become 'dislocated' once again in the bottom strip.

4. A PROPENSITY TO VENTRICULAR CAPTURE BEATS

The relatively slow idionodal rate (when compared with the more rapid rates of extrasystolic A-V nodal tachycardia) results in a relatively long cycle length or diastolic period relative to the refractory period. This facilitates the opportunity for ventricular capture beats, since a sinus impulse that occurs during the end of the idionodal cycle will, under these circumstances, probably encounter responsive A-V nodal tissue, and be conducted to the ventricles. The rapid rate of the extrasystolic form of A-V nodal tachycardia results in a short cycle relative to the refractory period, and this militates against the occurrence of ventricular capture beats.

5. THE ABSENCE OF PACEMAKER PROTECTION

The absence of protection of the A-V nodal pacemaker in idionodal tachycardia is evident from:

A. The abolition of the idionodal tachycardia if and when the sinus rhythm accelerates and usurps control of the heart once again.

B. The 'dislocation' of the ectopic rhythm by a capture beat. The ectopic cycle is re-set by the capturing impulse, thereby indicating that the capturing impulse penetrated into the A-V nodal pacemaker site.

SIGNIFICANCE

The clinical significance of idionodal tachycardia is similar to that of idioventricular tachycardia (see page 193).

REFERENCE

1 PICK A. & DOMINGUEZ P. (1057) Nonparoxysmal A-V nodal tachycardia. *Circulation* **16,** 102.

Chapter 15
Ventricular Rhythms

VENTRICULAR EXTRASYSTOLES · VENTRICULAR TACHYCARDIA ·
VENTRICULAR FLUTTER · VENTRICULAR FIBRILLATION ·
VENTRICULAR PARASYSTOLE · VENTRICULAR ESCAPE

VENTRICULAR EXTRASYSTOLES

A ventricular extrasystole is due to the **premature** discharge of an **ectopic ventricular focus.** It has the following characteristics:

1. THE DISCHARGE IS PREMATURE

The ventricular extrasystole is premature and arises in the diastolic period of the preceding sinus beat. It is, therefore, recorded earlier than the next anticipated sinus beat (Figs. 157, 158, 159, 160 and 161).

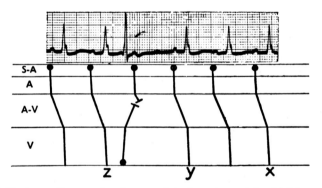

Fig. 157. Electrocardiogram showing a ventricular extrasystole which has discharged before the following sinus P wave. The P wave is recorded after the bizarre QRS complex and is seen superimposed on the S-T segment of the extrasystole. The compensatory pause is complete, i.e. the sum of the pre- and post-ectopic intervals (Z–Y) equals the sum of two consecutive sinus cycles (Y–X). Black dots indicate impulse origin.

2. THE QRS COMPLEX IS BIZARRE

The discharge arises in an ectopic focus and the course of depolarization is consequently abnormal. Furthermore, the impulse does not travel through specialized conduction tissue but through ordinary muscle tissue, which is relatively poor conducting medium. As a

179

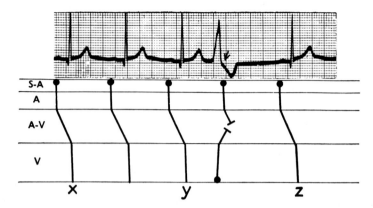

Fig. 158. Electrocardiogram (Standard lead II) showing a ventricular extrasystole. Note (*a*) the bizarre premature QRS complex of the extrasystole which occurs concomitantly with a sinus discharge; the P wave of this sinus discharge is thus largely hidden within the QRST complex of the extrasystole but may just be seen as a slight deformity (barely discernible) on the proximal part of the S-T segment (arrow); (*b*) the compensatory pause is complete, i.e. the sum of the pre- and post-ectopic intervals (Y–Z) is exactly equal to two consecutive sinus cycles (X–Y)—(see also Fig. 157).

result the QRS complex is bizarre-widened and slurred or notched (Fig. 158).

3. THERE ARE SECONDARY S-T SEGMENT AND T WAVE CHANGES

When the QRS complex is dominantly upright, the S-T segment is depressed and minimally convex-upward; and the T wave is inverted. When the QRS complex is dominantly downward, the S-T segment is elevated and minimally concave-upward; and the T wave is upright. These changes are secondary to the abnormal depolarization, and in themselves do not connote primary myocardial abnormality. These manifestations are similar to the secondary changes seen in classic right or left bundle branch block.

4. THE COUPLING INTERVAL IS CONSTANT

The coupling interval is the interval between the ectopic beat and the preceding sinus beat, and is constant for all extrasystoles arising from the same focus, i.e. extrasystoles of the same size and shape and presenting in the same lead of the same tracing. This is because the extrasystole is in some way related to, precipitated, or forced, by the preceding sinus beat.

5. RELATIONSHIP TO THE NEAR-SYNCHRONOUS SINUS P WAVE

(A) *The ventricular extrasystoles may be dissociated from, and have the following relationship to, the ensuing or near-synchronous sinus discharge*

(i) The ventricular extrasystole may manifest just before the following sinus discharge. When this occurs, the sinus P wave will be recorded after the bizarre QRS complex of the extrasystole and may be superimposed on the S-T segment of the extrasystole (Fig. 139).

(ii) The ventricular extrasystole may manifest at the same time as the following sinus discharge. When this occurs, the sinus P wave will be superimposed upon, or hidden within and thus masked by, the bizarre QRS complex of the extrasystole (Fig. 158).

(iii) The ventricular extrasystole, although premature, may manifest relatively late, i.e. immediately after the sinus discharge but before the sinus impulse reaches the ventricles (Fig. 159). The

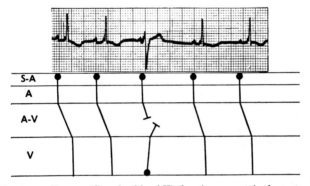

Fig. 159. Electrocardiogram (Standard lead II) showing a ventricular extrasystole which has discharged relatively late—an end-diastolic ventricular extrasystole, i.e. it occurs just after the following sinus discharge. The P wave of this sinus discharge is thus recorded just before the bizarre complex of the ventricular extrasystole (see also Fig. 162A).

dissociated sinus P wave is then recorded just before the bizarre QRS complex of the extrasystole. The 'P–R' interval is very short. This is known as an *end-diastolic ventricular extrasystole.*

In all the instances cited above (Figs. 157, 158 and 159), the sinus and extrasystolic impulses meet and interfere with each other in the A-V node, i.e. the sinus impulse is prevented from passing to the ventricles, and the ventricular impulse is prevented from passing to the atria.

At times, an end-diastolic ventricular extrasystolic impulse may invade the ventricles at the same time as the sinus impulse, thereby resulting in a ventricular fusion beat (see also Chapter 24, page 255).

(B) *Retrograde conduction of the ventricular extrasystole*

Occasionally, in the presence of a basic sinus bradycardia, or when the ventricular extrasystole is very premature, the extrasystolic discharge occurs long before the next scheduled sinus discharge.

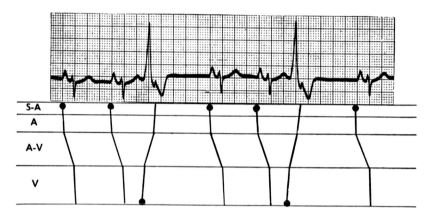

Fig. 160. Electrocardiogram (Standard lead II) showing ventricular extrasystoles with retrograde conduction to the atria. Note (*a*) an inverted P wave follows each extrasystole; (*b*) the inverted P wave is premature, i.e. it occurs earlier than the next anticipated sinus P wave (the normal P–P interval = 0.80 sec, the intervals between the inverted P wave and the preceding P wave = 0.68 sec). Large black dots indicate impulse origin.

Consequently, the ectopic impulse reaches the A-V node and atria *before* they have been activated by the sinus impulse. The ectopic impulse can then be conducted retrogradely to the atria and may even reach the S-A node and discharge it prematurely (Fig. 160). The bizarre QRS complex of the ventricular extrasystole is thus followed by a premature and 'retrograde'—usually inverted—P wave (compare A-V nodal extrasystole with retrograde conduction—page 159). See also section on Interpolated Ventricular Extrasystoles (page 183).

6. THE COMPENSATORY PAUSE

When the ventricular extrasystole is dissociated from the sinus impulse (described above in paragraphs 5 (i), (ii), (iii)), the ectopic impulse is unable to penetrate the A-V node retrogradely. The discharge of the S-A node is thus not interfered with and the S-A node is, in a sense, protected from the ectopic impulse. The sinus rhythm continues undisturbed, i.e. the next sinus impulse (the one following the dissociated beat) occurs on schedule. The pause following the extrasystole—the compensatory pause—is thus complete, i.e. it compensates exactly for the extrasystolic prematurity—the sum of the pre- and post-ectopic intervals (Y–Z in Figs. 157 and 158) is exactly equal to the sum of two consecutive sinus intervals (X–Y in Figs. 157 and 158).

With retrograde conduction of the ventricular extrasystole (described in (B) above), the sinus node is discharged prematurely by the ectopic impulse and the compensatory pause may, theoretically, be incomplete (compare sequence of events in atrial extrasystole.

7. THE 'RULE OF BIGEMINY'

Ventricular extrasystoles tend to follow long R–R intervals—the 'Rule of Bigeminy' (Langendorf, Pick & Winternitz, 1955[7]). A long cycle or R–R interval precipitates an ensuing ventricular extrasystole. This phenomenon is best seen during irregular rhythms, e.g. marked sinus arrhythmia or atrial fibrillation (Figs. 163 and 164). The compensatory pause of the extrasystole, in turn, constitutes another long R–R interval which tends to precipitate a further extrasystole. This process is thus self-perpetuating, resulting in bigeminal rhythm.

Not all ventricular extrasystoles obey this rule (Schamroth, 1965[10]).

Interpolated ventricular extrasystoles

An interpolated ventricular extrasystole is an, extrasystole which is, so-to-speak, 'sandwiched' between two conducted sinus beats (Fig. 161). It, therefore, occurs without a compensatory pause. Interpolated ventricular extrasystoles are nearly always associated with sinus bradycardia.

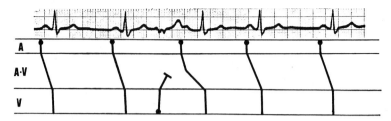

Fig. 161. Electrocardiogram showing an interpolated ventricular extrasystole. Note (*a*) the ventricular extrasystole is 'sandwiched' between two sinus beats; (*b*) there is no disturbance of sinus rhythm; (*c*) the P–R interval of the sinus beat following the extrasystole is longer than the P–R interval of the sinus beat preceding the extrasystole. Black dots indicate impulse origin.

MECHANISM

(*a*) The ventricular extrasystole occurs very early, i.e. at a time when the A-V node is still partially refractory; retrograde conduction of the ectopic impulse to the atria is, therefore, blocked within the A-V node.

(*b*) The following sinus beat occurs on time, but relatively late in relationship to the extrasystole; it thus finds the A-V node and ventricles sufficiently recovered to respond; nevertheless, owing to some retrograde penetration of the ectopic impulse into the A-V node, the lower, or penetrated, region of the A-V node is still partially refractory, and the following sinus beat is, therefore, conducted with delay through this region, resulting in a longer than usual P–R interval.

This is the commonest manifestation of concealed conduction. The actual retrograde penetration of the ectopic ventricular impulse into the A-V node is not manifest electrocardiographically, i.e. it is concealed. The event, however, is evident from a subsequent disturbance of conduction.

CHARACTERISTICS OF INTERPOLATED VENTRICULAR
EXTRASYSTOLES

1. They occur during slow sinus rhythm.
2. The extrasystole is 'sandwiched' between two sinus beats and there is no compensatory pause.
3. The sinus beat following the extrasystole has a longer P–R interval than the sinus beat preceding the extrasystole.

Extrasystolic ventricular bigeminy

Alternate ventricular extrasystoles, i.e. extrasystoles which occur after every other sinus beat, are the commonest cause of bigeminal rhythm (Fig. 162) and a frequent manifestation of digitalis intoxication.

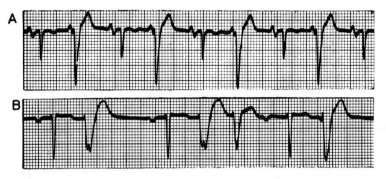

Fig. 162. Electrocardiogram (both tracings of lead V1) showing bigeminal rhythm due to alternate ventricular extrasystoles. (A) shows end-diastolic ventricular extrasystoles (compare Fig. 141). Note the constant coupling intervals. (B) shows an instance of ventricular trigeminy resulting from a pair of consecutive ventricular extrasystoles.

Multifocal or multiform ventricular extrasystoles

Extrasystoles that arise from different foci and consequently give rise to different QRS complexes are termed multifocal or multiform ventricular extrasystoles (Fig. 163).

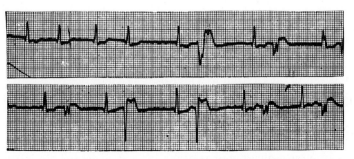

Fig. 163. Electrocardiogram (continuous strip of Standard lead II) showing (*a*) atrial fibrillation; (*b*) multiform ventricular extrasystoles. Note the first ventricular extrasystole follows a long R–R interval—the 'Rule of Bigeminy'.

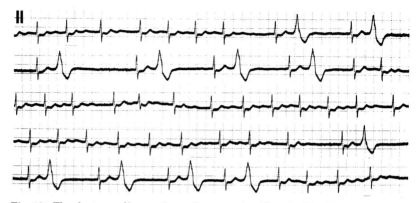

Fig. 164. The electrocardiogram (a continuous strip of Standard lead II) shows the following features: 1. *Atrial fibrillation*. This is reflected by the irregular baseline which is minimally distorted by the very fine, irregular and bizarre visible 'f' waves. There are no recognizable P waves. The ventricular response is irregular, resulting in cycles that vary from 0.60 sec to 1.24 sec. 2. *Digitalis effect*. The S-T segments reflect the mirror-image of a correction-mark configuration, connoting digitalis. 3. *Hypokalaemia*. This is reflected by a rather prominent U wave which is evident as a rounded deflection after the T wave. 4. *Ventricular extrasystoles*. These are reflected by the bizarre, premature and uniform QRS complexes. The ventricular extrasystoles alternate with the conducted fibrillation impulses giving rise to a bigeminal rhythm. The coupling intervals of these ventricular extrasystoles are constant and measure 0.46 sec. 5. *The 'Rule of Bigeminy'*. The precipitation of a ventricular extrasystole is favoured by a long preceding cycle of R–R interval. The first ventricular extrasystole in the top strip follows the longest R–R interval in that strip. The compensatory pause of this first ventricular extrasystole constitutes another long R–R interval which, in turn, favours the precipitation of a further ventricular extrasystole. The bigeminal rhythm thus tends to be perpetuated. A similar phenomenon is evident in the fourth strip. *Note*: The bigeminal rhythm ceases when the compensatory pause of the ventricular extrasystole shortens. This is evident at the end of the periods of bigeminal rhythm in the second and fifth strips.

Extrasystoles in pairs

When a ventricular ectopic focus discharges prematurely and twice in succession, the rhythm will manifest as a pair of extrasystoles, viz. a sinus beat followed by two extrasystoles (Figs. 162 and 165C).

Extrasystolic—paroxysmal—ventricular tachycardia

Three or more successive ventricular extrasystoles constitute an extrasystolic ventricular tachycardia—a paroxysmal tachycardia (Fig. 165).

SIGNIFICANCE OF VENTRICULAR EXTRASYSTOLES

Although isolated ventricular extrasystoles may occasionally be found in individuals without manifest heart disease their presence should always be viewed with suspicion.

Ventricular extrasystoles are always significant when associated with myocardial disease.

Multifocal ventricular extrasystoles and ventricular extrasystoles in pairs are *always* abnormal and usually indicative of serious myocardial disease.

Unifocal ventricular extrasystoles are usually indicative of cardiac disease if (a) they occur frequently, i.e. in 'crops' or 'showers', (b) they occur in bigeminal rhythm, (c) they occur in association with cardiac disease, (d) they occur in persons over 40 years of age or (e) they are precipitated by exercise.

Frequent ventricular extrasystoles, especially those occurring in pairs, often herald ventricular tachycardia or ventricular fibrillation.

The following schema is a rough but not necessarily absolute guide to the state of ectopic ventricular automaticity.

In the early stages of ectopic ventricular irritability, or automaticity, only occasional extrasystoles are evident (Fig. 165, strip A). Further evolution, i.e. increasing ventricular automaticity, is manifested by (a) ventricular extrasystoles in bigeminal rhythm (strip B), (b) extrasystoles in pairs (strip C) and (c) ventricular tachycardia (strip D).

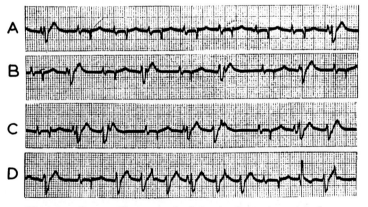

Fig. 165. Electrocardiogram illustrating both levels of ectopic ventricular irritability. A = occasional ventricular extrasystoles. B = extrasyctoles in bigeminal rhythm. C = extrasystoles in pairs. D = paroxysmal ventricular tachycardia.

Ventricular extrasystoles complicating myocardial infarction worsen the prognosis.

Digitalis intoxication is the commonest cause of ventricular extrasystolic bigeminal rhythm and the advent of this rhythm during digitalis administration is an absolute indication to stop therapy. Digitalis intoxication will rarely, if ever, cause ventricular extrasystolic bigeminal rhythm in a normal heart.

VENTRICULAR EXTRASYSTOLES WITH VERY SHORT COUPLING INTERVALS: THE 'R ON T' PHENOMENON

A ventricular extrasystole may rarely occur with a very short coupling interval, and will consequently coincide with, and be superimposed upon, or near, the apex or the distal limb of the preceding T wave (Fig. 172). Ventricular extrasystoles with this marked prematurity reflect an ominous situation for they are then likely to occur during the 'vulnerable phase' of the recovering ventricular myocardium and will consequently be prone to precipitate ventricular fibrillation.

Ventricular extrasystoles with such short coupling intervals almost invariable occur in the context of the acute insult to the heart such as acute myocardial infarction.

It should be stressed that a ventricular extrasystole which occurs with so short a coupling interval indicates that the refractory period of the myocardium, or part of the myocardium, has to be abnormally and pathologically shortened. And it is this abnormal shortening which is the basic underlying substrate for the vulnerability to ventricular fibrillation.

VENTRICULAR TACHYCARDIA

Ventricular tachycardia is due to the rapid discharge of an ectopic ventricular pacemaking focus. It may be defined as a series of three or more consecutive ventricular ectopic beats which are recorded in rapid succession. There are two principal forms:

    1. Extrasystolic Ventricular Tachycardia.
    2. Idioventricular Tachycardia.

EXTRASYSTOLIC VENTRICULAR TACHYCARDIA

Extrasystolic ventricular tachycardia is a series of three or more consecutive ventricular extrasystoles.

Electrocardiographic manifestation

1. BIZARRE QRS COMPLEXES

The QRS complexes have the characteristics of ventricular extrasystoles, i.e. they are bizarre, premature, and are recorded in rapid succession (Figs. 165, 166 and 167). The characteristics of the QRS form are considered further in Chapter 25.

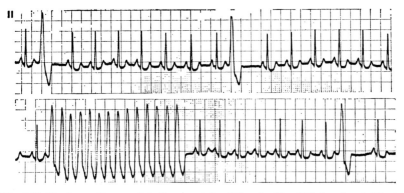

Fig. 166. Electrocardiogram (continuous strip of Standard lead II) showing: 1. Sinus tachycardia, reflected by the normal P-QRS-T complexes recorded in rapid succession; rate = 120 beats per minute. 2. Ventricular extrasystoles, reflected by the bizarre, isolated, and premature QRS complexes. A paroxysm of extrasystolic ventricular tachycardia, reflected by the series of 14 consecutive ventricular extrasystoles recorded in very rapid succession.

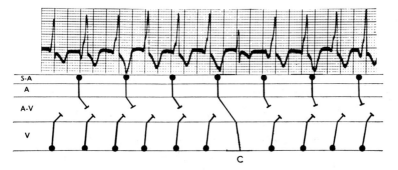

Fig. 167. Electrocardiogram illustrating paroxysmal ventricular tachycardia. Note (*a*) the bizarre QRS complexes of the ectopic discharge which are completely dissociated from the P waves of the sinus discharge; (*b*) the complex labelled C represents a capture beat—it is near-normal in configuration and is preceded by a P wave (seen superimposed on the preceding T wave).

2. A-V DISSOCIATION

The ectopic ventricular rhythm and the sinus rhythm may be dissociated. When this occurs, the sinus impulses and the ectopic ventricular impulses meet within the A-V node and impede or interfere with each other's mutual progress (compare with the dissociated form of ventricular extrasystoles—Section A on page 181). The **P waves therefore bear no relationship to the QRS complexes** (Figs. 165, 166 and 167).

3. RETROGRADE V-A CONDUCTION

The ectopic ventricular impulses may, at times, be conducted retrogradely to the atria (Fig. 228). Activation of the atria is then effected retrogradely by the ectopic ventricular impulses, and the bizarre QRS complexes are then followed by 'retrograde' P′ waves: P′ waves which are inverted in Standard leads II and III, and lead AVF, and which are pointed and dominantly positive in lead V1.

Note: Every QRS complex is followed by an abnormal P′ wave but it is often difficult, and at times impossible, to tell (*a*) whether such P′ waves are the result of ventricular tachycardia with retrograde conduction, or (*b*) whether they represent atrial paroxysmal tachycardia with phasic aberrant ventricular conduction (see page 266). The diagnosis can only be made with certainty when the beginning of a paroxysm is recorded: in the case of a ventricular tachycardia, the abnormal P′ wave will *follow* the first bizarre QRS complex, whereas in atrial paroxysmal tachycardia with phasic aberrant ventricular conduction, the abnormal P′ wave will *precede* the first bizarre QRS complex (Fig. 227).

4. CAPTURE BEATS

When the sinus rhythm and the ventricular rhythm are dissociated, their impulses meet and interfere with each other's mutual progress within the A-V node. In other words, the A-V node is in a state of almost constant refractoriness due to prior penetration by either the sinus or ectopic impulses. Occasionally, however, with critical timing, and especially during relatively slow ventricular tachycardia, a sinus impulse may reach the A-V node during a non-refractory phase, i.e. just after a period of absolute refractoriness following partial retrograde penetration of the ectopic impulse into the A-V node. The sinus impulse can then be conducted to the ventricles and momentarily activate or capture the ventricles, i.e. for one beat only (Fig. 167). This conducted beat which occurs during the ectopic ventricular rhythm is known as a *capture beat*. The QRS complex of the capture beat is recognized because it resembles the conducted sinus beats during regular sinus rhythm. Furthermore, the capture beat is always related to a preceding sinus P wave (see also section on interference-dissociation—page 251). A capture beat, whose configuration differs from the QRS configuration of the basic ventricular tachycardia, is one of the more reliable diagnostic pointers to the ventricular origin of the basic tachycardia (see Chapter 25). Not infrequently, the ventricular capture is only partial: the sinus and ectopic ventricular impulses invade the ventricles synchronously, resulting in a ventricular fusion beat (see Chapter 24).

5. VENTRICULAR FUSION

At times, the capturing (sinus) impulse may invade the ventricles concomitantly with the ectopic ventricular impulse. When this occurs, each impulse will activate part of the ventricles, and the resulting QRS complex will have a configuration that is in between that of the 'pure' sinus beat (seen during uncomplicated sinus rhythm) and the 'pure' ectopic beat. This combination or summation beat is known as a *ventricular fusion beat* (see also section on ventricular fusion beats in ventricular parasystole—page 202). A ventricular fusion beat is the most reliable diagnostic pointer to the ventricular origin of the basic tachycardia.

SIGNIFICANCE

Extrasystolic—paroxysmal—ventricular tachycardia is usually associated with advanced myocardial disease, most commonly ischaemic heart disease, and is frequently a manifestation of digitalis intoxication.

IDIOVENTRICULAR TACHYCARDIA[11, 12]
(syn. Accelerated Ventricular Rhythm)

The heart has many potential pacemaking cells which are situated in the S-A node, the atria, the A-V node, and the ventricles. Only one of these pacemaking cells—the pacemaker with the highest automaticity or discharge rate—is, however, in control of the heart. This is because its impulses reach the slower potential subsidiary pacemakers, and abolish or discharge their immature impulses before they have the time or opportunity to reach maturity and 'fire'. The subsidiary pacemaking centres thus enjoy *no protection* from the impulses of the fastest pacemaker; and it is this which ensures that only one pacemaker is normally in control of the heart.

The inherent automaticity of the S-A node and the potential subsidiary pacemakers may, under certain circumstances, become enhanced. When, for example, the inherent automaticity of the S-A node is enhanced, the rhythm manifests as a sinus tachycardia. The inherent rate of the A-V nodal pacemaker—the idionodal rhythm— may be similarly enhanced and, if the enhanced A-V nodal rate exceeds the sinus rate, the A-V nodal rhythm becomes manifest. This accelerated idionodal rhythm is known as *idionodal tachycardia.* An inherent idioventricular rhythm may be similarly enhanced result- ing in an *idioventricular tachycardia.*

If an enhanced idionodal rhythm or an enhanced idioventricular rhythm is to become manifest, it is clear that a disproportionate or differential enhancing influence must be present; an influence that affects the idionodal rhythm or the idioventricular rhythm to a greater degree than the sinus rhythm, or, an influence that only affects a particular pacemaker.

Electrocardiographic criteria

The diagnosis of idioventricular tachycardia is based on the follow- ing manifestations (Figs. 169 and 170):

1. Evidence of ventricular origin, e.g. bizarre QRS complexes, ventricular fusion beats (see also page 268).
2. A *relatively* rapid idioventricular rate. The idioventricular rhythm is usually accelerated to the same rate-range as that of the sinus rhythm, i.e. in the range of 70 to 80 beats per minute.
3. *A propensity to A-V dissociation and capture beats.* Since idioven- tricular tachycardia usually occurs in approximately the same rate-range as that of sinus rhythm, the two rhythms commonly discharge simultaneously (Fig. 168). A-V dissociation is, therefore, a common occurrence. Furthermore, capture beats—both complete and incomplete (fusion beats)—are also very common. This is due to the *relatively* slow rate of the idioventricular tachycardia; the relatively long cycle permits adequate recovery time and, thereby, a greater opportunity for capture. With very fast rates, as occurs in extrasystolic ventricular tachycardia, the refractory period frequently occupies the whole or practically the whole ectopic

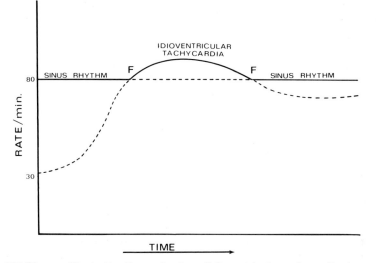

Fig. 168. Diagram illustrating the mechanism of idioventricular tachycardia. A potential idioventricular rhythm (dotted line) is enhanced until it exceeds the sinus rhythm and becomes manifest as an idioventricular tachycardia. At points F both the sinus and idioventricular rhythms will be the same rate, thereby resulting in ventricular fusion beats.

cycle, and the opportunity for capture is consequently minimal or absent.

Since idioventricular tachycardia becomes manifest when its rate equals the sinus rate, the ectopic rhythm usually begins with several consecutive fusion beats—incomplete capture beats (Fig. 169). And since the two rhythms tend to fluctuate within the same narrow range, the ectopic rhythm tends to terminate with several successive fusion complexes.

4. *The absence of pacemaker protection.* The ectopic pacemaker has no protection. This is evident from the abolition of the ectopic rhythm if and when the sinus rhythm regains its dominance. This is in contrast to ventricular parasystole where the ectopic rhythm is never abolished by a faster sinus rhythm (see page 201).

SIGNIFICANCE

Idioventricular tachycardia is the expression of *non-specific enhancement* of a pacemaker and may, for example, be associated with such non-specific 'activity' as *fever* and acute carditis. It is not infre-

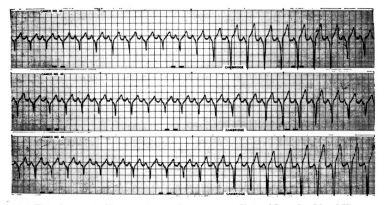

Fig. 169. The electrocardiogram (a continuous recording of Standard lead II) was recorded from a 66-year-old man with acute inferior myocardial infarction, and shows: 1. *Sinus tachycardia.* The P–P intervals measure 0.56 sec., reflecting a rate of 107 beats per minute. 2. *Idioventricular tachycardia.* This is represented by the bizarre QRS complexes at the end of each strip. These bizarre QRS complexes are not related to the P waves which occur just before, and are sometimes superimposed upon or hidden within, the proximal part of the bizarre QRS complexes. This reflects the presence of A-V dissociation. The R–R intervals measure 0.56 sec., representing a rate of 107 beats per minute—a ventricular tachycardia. The 'pure' ectopic complex is represented, for example, by the seven bizarre QRS complexes at the end of the top strip. The two QRS complexes preceding and the two QRS complexes following this period of idioventricular tachycardia have a configuration that is in between that of the 'pure' ectopic beat and the 'pure' sinus beat. These are ventricular fusion complexes. Every period of ectopic ventricular rhythm begins and ends with ventricular fusion complexes. Ventricular fusion complexes may also be seen during the periods of dominant sinus rhythm, e.g. the 6th, 7th and 8th QRS complexes in the top strip are slightly modified, reflecting partial ventricular fusion.

quently associated with the administration of digitalis and is a common manifestation in acute myocardial infarction; commoner, in fact, than extrasystolic ventricular tachycardia.

As with sinus tachycardia, the rhythm itself rarely requires any active treatment. It is not a sudden precipitous, dramatic event, and is unlikely to precipitate ventricular fibrillation. Since it is usually in the same rate-range as that of the normal sinus rhythm, it rarely causes haemodynamic embarrassment. If the loss of atrial drive becomes significant (a rare event) the ectopic ventricular rhythm may be overdriven by accelerating the sinus rate with atropine. It is doubtful whether it is ever necessary to resort to electrical over-driving or the use of cardio-suppressive drugs such as lidocaine.

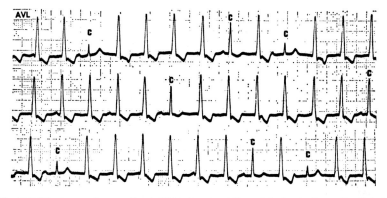

Fig. 170. Electrocardiogram (lead AVL) showing *idioventricular tachycardia*. This is reflected by the bizarre QRS complexes which are recorded at a rate of 104 beats per minute, and which bear no relationship to the P waves of the sinus rhythm. The rhythm is complicated by frequent capture beats (labelled C): the momentary conduction to, and capture of, the ventricles by the sinus impulse. Some of these capture beats are incomplete, i.e. the sinus impulse invades the ventricles concomitantly with the ventricular impulse, each activating part of the ventricles. This results in a ventricular fusion complex, a complex whose configuration is in between that of the 'pure' sinus beat and the 'pure' ectopic beat. The configuration of these partial capture beats varies and depends upon the relative contribution of each impulse to ventricular activation. When the contribution from the ectopic ventricular impulse is dominant, the ventricular fusion complex resembles the 'pure' ectopic beat, e.g. eighth QRS complex in the top strip and the last QRS complex in the middle strip. When the contribution from the sinus impulse is greater, the QRS complex will tend to resemble the 'pure' sinus beat, e.g. the third and tenth complexes in the top strip, and the second and eleventh QRS complexes in the bottom strip.

VENTRICULAR FLUTTER

Ventricular flutter is the expression of:

1. *A very rapid and regular ectopic ventricular discharge.*

2. *Grossly abnormal intraventricular conduction.* The QRS and T deflections are very wide and bizarre—one merging with the other—so that it is difficult to define or separate the QRS complex, S-T segment and T wave. This results in the appearance of a continuous sine-like wave-form (Fig. 171).

Note: This bizarre sine-like wave-form may result from the abnormal intraventricular conduction alone. The appearance of ventricular flutter may thus occur at rates similar to that of extrasystolic ventricular tachycardia.

Co-ordinated activation and consequent haemodynamic contrac-

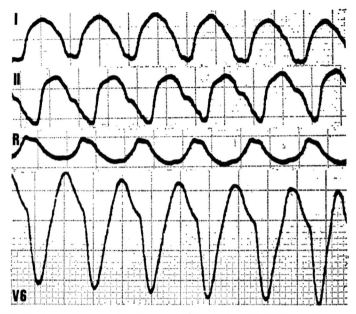

Fig. 171. Electrocardiogram showing ventricular flutter. The QRS complexes are very wide, bizarre, and blend imperceptibly with the T waves so that a separation of the two is difficult. The effect is that of a continuous 'sine-like' wave form (best seen in Standard lead I).

tion is still present. However, the change from extrasystolic tachycardia to ventricular flutter is associated with a fall in blood pressure and cardiac output (Smirk, Nolla-Panades & Wallis, 1964[14]).

Ventricular flutter is uncommon. Few examples are recorded since the condition usually progresses or changes rapidly to ventricular fibrillation.

Ventricular flutter differs from ventricular fibrillation by the uniformity, constancy, regularity, and relatively large amplitude of the deflections. The deflections of ventricular fibrillation are small and completely chaotic and irregular.

It may well be that ventricular flutter and extrasystolic ventricular tachycardia are expressions of the same mechanism. Their separation may, nevertheless, serve a useful purpose, since a diagnosis of ventricular flutter immediately connotes a very rapid ventricular rate and/or grossly abnormal intraventricular conduction, and reflects an ominous clinical state with a drop in blood pressure and a low cardiac output.

MULTIFORM VENTRICULAR FLUTTER:
'TORSADES DE POINTES'

Ventricular flutter may present with multiform QRS complexes, a manifestation which has been termed 'torsades de pointes'[2, 3, 9] (Fig. 184). The QRS complexes tend to be bizarre, multiform, and have sharply pointed apices or nadirs. The QRS form and axis undulates. Thus, the sharp points of the QRS complex may, for a short period of a few seconds, be directed upwards, to be followed for a short period of a few seconds, by a change in QRS contour where the sharp points are directed downwards. Hence the term 'torsades de pointes' which means a torsion of points. The rhythm is often interspersed with a single isolated normal or near-normal QRS complex. These not infrequently occur during the transition from upward to downward directed points of the QRS configuration (Fig. 184). It must, however, be emphasized that torsades de pointes is merely a descriptive term and does not define a mechanism. The basic mechanism should therefore be stated and further qualified, if desired, by the descriptive term. Thus: multiform ventricular flutter—torsades de pointes.

This form of ventricular flutter is particularly likely to complicate advanced and third degree A-V block, and is frequently associated with syncopal attacks. The complicating syncopal attacks result in marked prolongation of the Q–Tc and the 'giant T wave inversion syndrome' (page 213). Because of the marked prolongation of the Q–T interval, complicating ventricular extrasystoles with normal or relatively long coupling intervals, and which would normally fall well clear of the T wave, are now likely to occur on or near the apex of the 'giant' T wave, i.e. during the vulnerable phase of ventricular repolarization. They are consequently likely to precipitate the ventricular tachyarrhythmia (Fig. 184). In other words, the Q–T lengthening favours the 'R on T' phenomenon with normal or relatively long coupling intervals. As indicated above, the 'giant' T wave—the part expression of the prolonged Q–T interval—is the expression of a recent syncopal attack. It may, however, be difficult to determine whether such a syncopal attack is due to a period of ventricular asystole from the advanced A-V block, or the complicating ventricular flutter.

The association of the advanced A-V block with multiform ventricular flutter may be an expression of severe coronary artery disease, hypokalaemia, hypomagnasaemia or quinidine therapy.[9]

VENTRICULAR FIBRILLATION

Ventricular fibrillation is the expression of *chaotic, inco-ordinated, ventricular depolarization.* The bi-ventricular chamber is electrophysiologically 'fragmented' into a mosaic of milling tissue islets in various stages of recovery and excitation. The co-ordinated ventricular activation and the resulting co-ordinated muscle contraction is lost. The haemodynamic pumping action of the heart, therefore, ceases and death ensues within minutes unless defibrillation is instituted. The electrocardiogram manifests with *completely irregular, chaotic and deformed deflections of* varying height, width and shape (Fig. 172). Regular wave-forms such as P waves, QRS complexes, S-T segments and T waves cannot be identified.

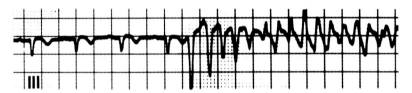

Fig. 172. Electrocardiogram showing sinus rhythm for the first 4 beats. These beats reflect the fully evolved phase of inferior wall myocardial infarction. The fourth beat is followed by a very premature ventricular extrasystole which occurs near the apex of the T wave of the sinus beat—the 'R on T' phenomenon. This precipitates ventricular fibrillation. Note the complete irregularity in the size, shape and rhythm of the electrocardiographic deflection. There is no recognizable pattern.

AETIOLOGY

Ventricular fibrillation is usually a terminal event, and is frequently associated with ischaemic heart disease, especially acute myocardial infarction. It may accompany quinidine and digitalis intoxication, especially when digitalis intoxication is associated with hypokalaemia, and advanced heart disease. It occurs characteristically with hypothermia when the body temperature drops below 28°C.

Ventricular fibrillation is probably the cause of death in cases of the Jervell–Lange-Nielsen syndrome[6]: a syndrome characterized by congenital deafness, syncopal attacks, prolonged Q–T interval and sudden death.

PRIMARY AND SECONDARY VENTRICULAR FIBRILLATION

The concept of primary and secondary ventricular fibrillation was introduced by Meltzer & Kitchell in 1966.[8]

Primary ventricular fibrillation refers to ventricular fibrillation that occurs in a patient without pre-existing or associated hypotension (systolic blood pressure less than 100 mmHg) or cardiac failure.

Secondary ventricular fibrillation refers to ventricular fibrillation that occurs in a patient who has lost a vital function, e.g. a patient with hypotension, respiratory failure or cardiac failure.

Primary ventricular fibrillation responds relatively well to electrical defibrillation, and resuscitation is usually successful. Secondary ventricular fibrillation is agonal and resuscitation usually fails.

MECHANISM

The predisposition to, and development of, ventricular fibrillation is favoured by the co-incidence of two fundamental events:

1. *An advanced physiological asymmetry of the biventricular chamber*. This is a non-homogeneous state of myocardial refractoriness—a dispersion of refractoriness. This asymmetrical state can only come about as a result of severe, and usually advanced, diseased processes such as myocardial infarction. These advanced disease processes result in local oxygen lack, local glucose deficiency and local ionic changes such as calcium excess, potassium excess or sodium deficiency.

2. *Premature or rapid repetitive stimulation of the asymmetrical chamber*. Rapid and or premature stimulation of the asymmetrical bi-ventricular chamber may aggravate the out-of-phase state, and thereby precipitate fibrillation.

The sources of such premature or rapid stimulation are:

A. *Ventricular extrasystoles*

Ventricular extrasystoles may precipitate ventricular fibrillation (Fig. 172). Ventricular fibrillation is often preceded by a ventricular extrasystole with a very short coupling interval; a coupling interval reflected by a ventricular extrasystole that occurs co-incidentally with the apex of the preceding T wave—the 'R on T' phenomenon.[1, 4, 5, 13, 15] This represents the vulnerable phase of ventricular excitability, and an extrasystolic impulse occurring during this phase is likely to precipitate ventricular fibrillation.

B. *Very rapid ventricular tachycarrhythmias*

Very rapid ventricular tachyarrhythmias such as extrasystolic ventricular tachycardia or ventricular flutter frequently precede and predispose to ventricular fibrillation.

VENTRICULAR PARASYSTOLE

(This is discussed in Chapter 16.)

VENTRICULAR ESCAPE

(This is discussed in Chapter 22.)

REFERENCES

1 ANDRUS E. C., CARTER E. P. & WHEELER H. A. (1930) The refractory period of the normal beating dog's auricle: with a note on the occurrence of auricular fibrillation following a single stimulus. *J. exp. Med.* **51**, 357.
2 BROCHIER M., MOTTE G. & FAUCHIER J. P. (1972) Tachycardie ventriculaire en torsades de pointes. *Actual Cardiol. Vasc.* **6**, 171.
3 DESSERTENNE F. (1966) La tachycardie ventriculaire a deux foyers opposes variable. *Arch. Mal. Coeur*, **59**, 263.
4 DOLARA A. (1967) Early premature ventricular beats with repetitive ventricular fibrillation. *Am. Heart J.* **74**, 332.
5 GUTIERREZ M. R., CHANGFOOT G. H. & PERETZ D. I. (1968) Significance of T wave interruption by premature beats as a cause of sudden death. *Canad. Med. Ass. J.* **98**, 144.
6 JERVELL A. & LANGE-NIELSEN F. (1957) Congenital deaf-mutism, functional heart disease with prolongation of the Q-T interval and sudden death. *Am. Heart J.* **54**, 59.
7 LANGENDORF R., PICK A. & WINTERNITZ M. (1955) Mechanisms of intermittent ventricular bigeminy. *Circulation* **11**, 422.
8 MELTZER L. E. & KITCHELL J. R. (1966) The incidence of arrhythmias associated with acute myocardial infarction. *Prog. Cardiovasc. Dis.* **9**, 50.
9 MOTTE G., COUMEL P., ABITBOL G., DESSERTENNE G. & SLAMA R. (1970) Le syndrome QT long et syncopes par 'torsades de pointes'. *Arch. Mal. Coeur.* **63**, 831.
10 SCHAMROTH L. (1965) Concealed extrasystoles and the Rule of Bigeminy. *Cardiologia* **46**, 51.
11 SCHAMROTH L. (1968) Idioventricular tachycardia. *J. Electrocardiol.* **1**, 205.
12 SCHAMROTH L. (1969) Idioventricular tachycardia. Editorial. *Dis. Chest* **56**, 466.
13 SMIRK F. H. & PALMER D. G. (1960) A myocardial syndrome with particular reference to the occurrence of sudden death and of premature systoles interrupting antecedent T waves. *Am. J. Cardiol.* **6**, 620.
14 SMIRK F. H., NOLLA-PANADES J. & WALLIS T. (1964) Experimental ventricular flutter and paroxysmal tachycardia. *Amer. J. Cardiol.* **14**, 79.
15 WIGGERS C. J. & WEGRIA R. (1940) Ventricular fibrillation due to single localised induction and condensor shocks applied during the vulnerable phase of ventricular systole. *Am. J. Physiol.* **128**, 500.

Chapter 16
Parasystole

It is a fundamental law of cardiac physiology that the dominant or fastest pacemaker determines the heart rate. All other subsidiary or slower potential pacemakers are prematurely discharged by the impulses from the dominant pacemaker (see also page 201).

This is because the many natural pacemaking cells in the heart enjoy no protection from each other's impulses, and their electrical charges are therefore vulnerable to dissipation by each other's impulses. Thus, the impulses of the fastest pacemaker—usually the S-A node—reach the slower potential subsidiary pacemakers before they have an opportunity to 'fire', and discharge or abolish their immature impulses prematurely. The sinus pacemaker so-to-speak 'silences' or dominates the slower subsidiary pacemakers. Occasionally, however, a subsidiary pacemaking centre acquires the property of *protection*, a property that protects it completely from the impulses of the fastest pacemaker.

This protective mechanism is situated in the *vicinity of the ectopic focus* and is *operative all the time, viz. throughout the ectopic cycle, i.e. during its refractory phase as well as its non-refractory phase.* When this occurs, the impulses of the faster sinus pacemaker cannot penetrate into the ectopic pacemaking focus which, as a result, is able to discharge at its own inherent, usually slower, rate. Although the sinus impulses cannot penetrate into the ectopic pacemaking focus, the ectopic impulses are, nevertheless, able to leave the focus and activate the surrounding myocardium if and when the surrounding myocardium is responsive following prior activation by the sinus impulse. The protection is thus in the form of a uni-directional block (entrance block—exit conduction) which is situated within the immediate vicinity of the pacemaking cell.

The commonest and least complex form of parasystole is ventricular parasystole. An ectopic ventricular pacemaker that is so protected is able to discharge unhindered by the impulses of the dominant sinus pacemaker. Its discharge is independent of the sinus pacemaker, and bears no relation to the rate or rhythm of the sinus pacemaker. Two pacemakers then co-exist in the heart, each discharging at its own inherent and independent rate, and each activating the heart when it finds the myocardium in a responsive state. The two pacemakers so-to-speak co-exist as commensals, and the resulting arrhythmia is known as parasystole. **Parasystole is thus a form of dual rhythm wherein two pacemakers concurrently and independently govern the rhythm of the heart.**

ELECTROCARDIOGRAPHIC CHARACTERISTICS

1. VARYING COUPLING INTERVALS

The coupling interval is the interval between the ectopic beat and the preceding sinus beat. With ventricular extrasystoles the ectopic beat is in some way forced or precipitated by the preceding sinus beat (Chapter 13); the ectopic beats will thus bear a constant relation to the preceding sinus beats, i.e. the coupling intervals are constant. In parasystole the ectopic pacemaker is autonomous and beats independently of the sinus pacemaker; the two pacemakers beat asynchronously and consequently they have no relationship to each other, i.e. the coupling interval is usually different with each ectopic beat (Fig. 174). Marked variation of the coupling intervals is usually the cardinal sign which alerts the electrocardiologist to the possible presence of a parasystolic mechanism.

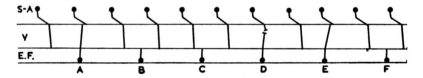

Fig. 173. Diagram illustrating ventricular parasystole. The S-A node discharges regularly but its impulse is unable to penetrate the protected ectopic ventricular focus (E.F.). The ectopic focus is thus not disturbed by the sinus rhythm and discharges regularly but at a slower rate than the S-A node. Ectopic impulses B, C and F find the surrounding myocardium refractory as a result of prior stimulation by the sinus impulse; these discharges are, therefore, confined to the ectopic focus and are not manifested electrocardiographically. Ectopic impulses A, D and E find the myocardium non-refractory and thus invade the myocardium, becoming manifest. They bear no relationship to their preceding sinus beats; as is evidenced by the marked variation of the coupling intervals. As the ectopic discharge is regular, the longer manifest interectopic interval—A–D—must be a simple multiple—3 times the basic ectopic cycle length of the shortest manifest interectopic interval D–E. D is a fusion complex.

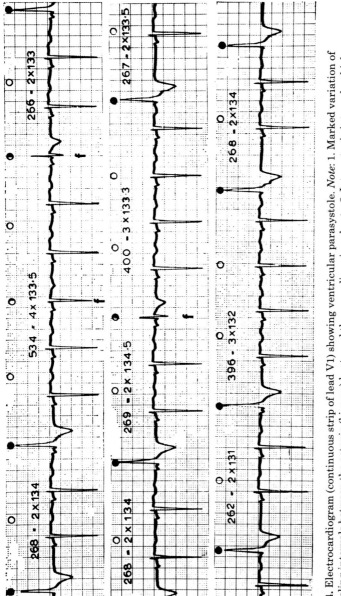

Fig. 174. Electrocardiogram (continuous strip of lead V1) showing ventricular parasystole. *Note:* 1. Marked variation of the coupling intervals between the ectopic (bizarre) beats and the preceding sinus beats. 2. Interectopic intervals which are all in multiples or near-multiples of 1.33 sec. 3. Fusion complexes (labelled f). 4. Black dots indicate manifest ectopic discharges. 5. Open circles indicate non-manifest ectopic discharges, reflecting the ectopic cycle length of 1.33 sec, as calculated from the longer interectopic intervals. 6. Half-open circles indicate fusion beats.

2. MATHEMATICALLY RELATED INTERECTOPIC INTERVALS

In parasystole some of the ectopic discharges are not manifest since they occur when the ventricles are refractory following activation by the sinus pacemaker. However, the ectopic pacemaker discharges regularly whether its impulses are able to activate the ventricles or not, and thus the longer interectopic intervals—the intervals between manifest ectopic discharges—are multiples of the shortest interectopic interval (Figs. 173 and 174).

3. FUSION BEATS (ALSO KNOWN AS SUMMATION OR COMBINATION BEATS)

As the two pacemakers in parasystole discharge at their own inherent rates, *occasional*, fortuitous, synchronous or near-synchronous discharge may occur. There will then be simultaneous invasion of the ventricular musculature by both impulses, each activating part of the ventricles. The resulting QRS complex has a configuration intermediate between the 'pure' sinus beat, and the 'pure' ventricular beat. The resulting summation or combination complex is known as a **fusion beat** (Figs. 173 and 174). The characteristics of ventricular fusion complexes are considered further on page 255.

SIGNIFICANCE

Parasystole is a relatively uncommon arrhythmia. It may occur with myocardial disease and in association with digitalis administration; but may also occur in normal individuals. There is no specific treatment. The treatment is that of the underlying condition.

SECTION 3
DISORDERS OF IMPULSE CONDUCTION

Sino-Atrial (S-A) Block
Atrioventricular (A-V) Block
Reciprocal Rhythm
The Supraventricular Tachycardias
The Wolff-Parkinson-White Syndrome

Chapter 17
Sino-Atrial (S-A) Block

In S-A block the sinus impulse is blocked *within* the S-A junction, i.e. the junction between the S-A node and the surrounding atrial myocardium. As a result, neither atrial nor ventricular activation takes place; no P wave or QRS complex is recorded, i.e. a *complete cardiac cycle so to speak 'drops out'* (Fig. 175). This is a form of exit block since the impulse cannot exit from its pacemaker site. S-A

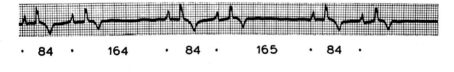

84 · 164 · 84 · 165 · 84 ·

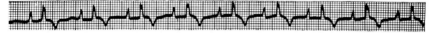

Fig. 175. *Top strip*: Electrocardiogram (Standard lead II) showing: 1. First degree A-V block. The P–R intervals measure 0.25 sec. 2. 3:2 S-A block. The P waves are distributed in a bigeminal grouping of long and short intervals. The relatively short P–P intervals of 0.84 sec alternate with intervals of 1.65 sec—almost twice the cycle length of the shorter interval. This indicates that the long interval is due to the omission of a complete P-QRS complex. Every third sinus impulse is blocked at the S-A junction resulting in a 3:2 S-A block. This causes a bigeminal rhythm.

Bottom strip: This was recorded after the administration of atropine. The S-A block is abolished and this is associated with a slight increase in the sinus rate.

205

block usually occurs irregularly and unpredictably as isolated instances. Very rarely, the block may occur at regular intervals, e.g. regular 2:1 S-A block. This resembles the slow regular rhythm of sinus bradycardia; the diagnosis can only be established when, in contrast to the gradual acceleration of sinus bradcycardia, the rate suddenly doubles with effort or atropine.

Following S-A block, the subsequent beat may be a normal sinus beat (Fig. 175), an A-V nodal escape beat (Fig. 139), or a ventricular escape beat (Fig. 140).

Note: In second-degree S-A block, *neither* the P wave *nor* the QRS complex is recorded at the moment of block; whereas in second-degree A-V block, *all* P waves are recorded but the P wave of the blocked beat is *not* followed by a QRS complex.

SIGNIFICANCE

S-A block is rare, but is found in the same conditions as marked sinus bradycardia or sinus arrhythmia. It occurs in young vagotonic individuals, particularly athletes, and also with digitalis administration. It is not infrequently associated with uraemia and occasionally with hypokalaemia. It may be an expression of Structural Nodal Disease, the so-called Sick Sinus Syndrome (see Chapter 26).

Chapter 18
Atrioventricular (A-V) Block

Atrioventricular (A-V) block is characterized by a **delay or interruption in conduction** of the atrial impulse through the specialized A-V conducting system: the A-V node and the bundle of His.
There are three degrees:
1. **First-degree A-V block:** a delay in conduction.
2. **Second-degree A-V block:** intermittent interruption of conduction.
3. **Third-degree A-V block:** complete or permanent interruption of conduction.

First- and second-degree A-V block are often referred to as *partial* or *incomplete A-V block*. A-V block is often loosely called heart block. This term, however, could have a wider meaning and embrace all forms of heart block, viz. sino-atrial block, atrioventricular block and intraventricular block. It is, therefore, best to refer to the form of block more specifically as A-V block.

FIRST-DEGREE A-V BLOCK
(Prolonged P–R Interval)

First-degree A-V block is a *delay* in conduction through the conducting system. It is reflected by a *prolonged P–R interval*. The P–R interval (sometimes referred to as the P–Q interval) is measured from the *beginning of the P wave* to the *beginning of the QRS complex*, irrespective of whether the QRS complex begins with q or an R wave (Figs. 176 and 241).

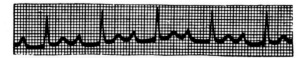

Fig. 176. Electrocardiogram (Standard lead II) showing sinus rhythm complicated by first-degree A-V block (prolonged P–R interval). The P–R interval, measured from the beginning of the P wave to the beginning of the QRS complex, equals 0.36 sec.

The P–R interval represents (*a*) the time taken for the impulse to travel from the S-A node to the A-V node (usually 0.03 sec) plus (*b*) the time taken for the impulse to travel through the A-V node, the bundle of His and the bundle branches to the ventricles; this represents by far the greater part of the P–R interval.

In first-degree A-V block the P–R interval is prolonged beyond the normal limit of 0.20 sec (beyond 0.18 sec in children). (Figs. 27, 140, 165, 175, 176 and 182.)

Note: In first-degree A-V block, *all* the P waves are followed by QRS complexes.

SIGNIFICANCE

First-degree A-V block is associated with *coronary artery disease, acute rheumatic carditis* and the *administration of digitalis and beta blockers.*

SECOND-DEGREE A-V BLOCK

Second-degree A-V block is characterized by an intermittent failure or interruption of A-V conduction. The sinus impulse, after leaving the S-A node and activating the atria to produce the P wave, is blocked within the A-V conducting system. The P wave is, therefore, *not* followed by a QRS complex and a ventricular beat is, so to speak, 'dropped'. Sinus rhythm complicated by second-degree A-V block

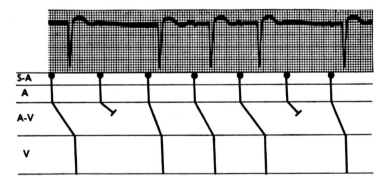

Fig. 177. Electrocardiogram (lead V3) showing sinus rhythm complicated by second-degree A-V block of the Wenckebach type. Note (*a*) that following the 'dropped' beat occasioned by a blocked sinus impulse, the P–R interval becomes progressively longer until another sinus impulse is blocked and a further beat is 'dropped'; (*b*) the atrial rhythm is regular and all the P waves are present; it is thus the QRS complex that is 'dropped'; (*c*) the fully evolved phase of anterior myocardial infarction.

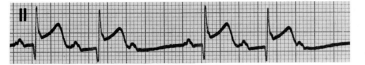

Fig. 178. Electrocardiogram (Standard lead II) showing the following features: A. The hyperacute phase of inferior wall myocardial infarction as evidenced by the tall R waves, the slope-elevation of the S-T segments and the tall and widened T waves; B. Sinus tachycardia. The P–P intervals measure 0.60 sec representing a rate of 100 per minute; C. 3:2 second-degree A-V block of the Wenckebach type. The first P–R interval measures 0.20 sec. The second P–R interval measures 0.29 sec. The third P wave is not followed by a QRS complex. This results in ventricular bigeminal rhythm.

(Courtesy of Catherine Marquard)

thus manifests with regularly occurring P waves, some of which are not followed by QRS complexes.

THE CONDUCTION RATIO

The sequences of second-degree A-V block may be expressed in the form of an A-V *conduction ratio*. This is the number of sinus impulses to the number of QRS complexes in any one sequence. A sequence begins with the first conducted sinus beat following a pause created by the 'dropped' beat and ending with, and including, the P wave of the ensuing blocked sinus impulse. See Figs. 178, 179, 180 and 181 for examples.

Note. Regular sinus rhythm complicated by 2:1 A-V block will result in a very slow regular ventricular rhythm (Fig. 187). Regular sinus rhythm complicated by 3:2 A-V block will result in a ventricular bigeminal rhythm (Figs 178 and 180). Variable—irregular—second-degree A-V block will result in an irregular ventricular rhythm (Fig. 179).

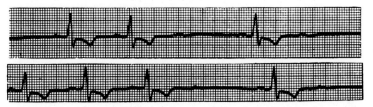

Fig. 179. Electrocardiogram (continuous strip of Standard lead II) showing sinus rhythm complicated by Type II second-degree A-V block. Note (*a*) beats are 'dropped' irregularly as a result of successive 3:2, 2:1, 4:3 and 2:1 A-V block; (*b*) the P–R interval is prolonged (0.26 sec) but is the same for all conducted beats; (*c*) the P wave is broad and notched reflecting a **P. mitrale.**

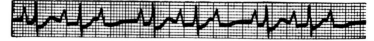

Fig. 180. Electrocardiogram (Standard lead II) showing: (*a*) Atrial tachycardia as reflected by the tall, pointed and abnormal P' waves which occur at a rate of 118 per minute and (*b*) bigeminal rhythm due to regularly recurring 3:2 A-V block of the Wenckebach type.

THE FORMS OF SECOND-DEGREE A-V BLOCK

The sinus impulses may be blocked at *regular or irregular intervals*, and the blocked impulse may be preceded by constant A-V conduction times—*constant P–R intervals*—or by a *progressive increase in P–R intervals*. These manifestations result in the following varieties of second degree A-V block.

1. Second-degree A-V block with the Wenckebach phenomenon
Synonym: Type I A-V block; Mobitz Type I A-V Block

In this type of second-degree A-V block, transmission through the conducting system becomes increasingly difficult until if fails completely and a beat is 'dropped'. The sequence begins with a normal or prolonged P–R interval; and with each successive beat the P–R interval lengthens until block of the supraventricular impulse occurs and a beat is 'dropped'. The pause occasioned by the 'dropped' beat allows the conducting system to recover and the sequence is then repeated (Figs. 177, 178 and 180). The defective mechanism giving rise to this form of second-degree A-V block is usually situated in the A-V node itself. This form of second-degree A-V block may be physiologi-

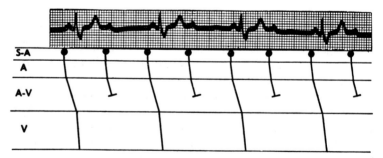

Fig. 181. Electrocardiogram showing sinus rhythm complicated by 2:1 A-V block. Note (*a*) the sinus rhythm is regular; (*b*) every second P wave is not followed by a QRS complex; (*c*) the consequent slow regular ventricular rate.

cal or pathological, but does not usually carry the adverse prognosis associated with the Type II A-V block (see below).

2. Second-degree A-V block with fixed A-V relationship
Synonym: Type II A-V block; Mobitz Type II A-V Block

In this form of second-degree A-V block, the P–R intervals of all the conducted supraventricular impulses are constant, i.e. there is no preceding progressive prolongation of the P–R intervals as occurs in the Wenckebach Phenomenon (Figs. 179 and 182). The associated QRS complex is frequently abnormal.

The lesion of this form of second-degree A-V block is usually situated in the bundle of His, and is always organic or pathological and carries an adverse prognosis, since it not infrequently progresses to complete A-V block.

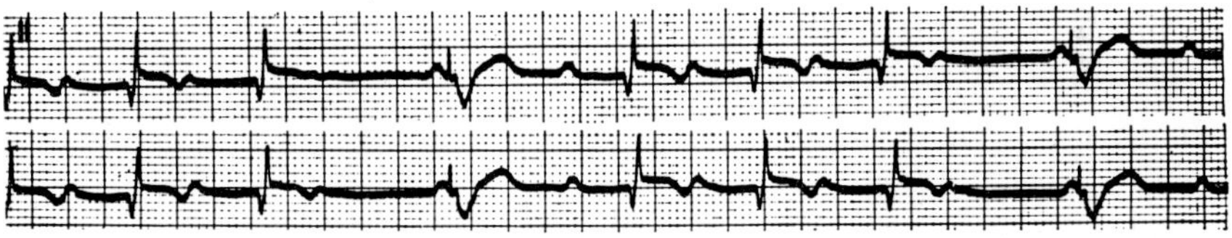

Fig. 182. Electrocardiogram (continuous strip of Standard lead II) showing: 1. The fully evolved phase of *acute myocardial infarction*. This is reflected by the pathological Q waves, raised, coved S-T segments and inverted T waves. 2. *Normal sinus rhythm.* 3. *First-degree A-V block.* The P–R intervals measure 0.36 sec. 4. *Type II second-degree A-V block.* There is intermittent interruption of conduction. The interruption is preceded by fixed or constant P–R intervals. 5. *Demand pacemaker escape.* The blocked sinus impulse is followed by the escape of an electrical demand pacemaker. Note the pacemaker artifact—the thin vertical line preceding each bizarre QRS complex. The pacemaker beat is dissociated from the near-synchronous P wave.

THE SIGNIFICANCE OF SECOND-DEGREE A-V BLOCK

Second-degree A-V block may occur in acute rheumatic carditis, in other forms of acute carditis, e.g. diphtheric carditis, in coronary artery disease and with digitalis administration.

Second-degree A-V block may be associated with fast supraventricular rhythms, e.g. atrial tachycardia and atrial flutter (Figs. 144 and 147). In these conditions, the presence of second-degree A-V block is usually physiological; the block only permits every second or third impulse to reach the ventricles, effectively slowing the ventricular rate and thereby acting as a 'protective' mechanism.

The degree and ratio of the block may fluctuate, e.g. a first-degree

A-V block may proceed to a second-degree A-V block, and a 2:1 ratio may change to a 4:3 ratio.

Atrial tachycardia with a varying 2:1 or 3:2 A-V block—so-called P.A.T. with block—is a common manifestation of digitalis intoxication (Fig. 144).

THIRD-DEGREE A-V BLOCK: COMPLETE A-V BLOCK

Third-degree A-V block is characterized by a complete or permanent interruption of A-V conduction, i.e. all the supraventricular impulses are blocked within the conducting system. The ventricles are then activated by a subsidiary ectopic escape pacemaker situated in the A-V node below the block or within the ventricles. The atria are thus activated by one pacemaker—usually the sinus pacemaker, and the ventricles by another—an idionodal or idioventricular pacemaker. The two rhythms are independent and *asynchronous*. This results in the following manifestations:

1. *A-V dissociation*

The *P waves bear no relationship to the QRS complexes.*

2. *A slow ventricular rate*

The inherent rate of an idioventricular pacemaker is slow, and is usually in the range of 30 to 35 beats per minute. A pacemaker situated more proximally, i.e. within the bundle of His, has a slightly faster inherent discharge rate, and is usually in the range of 35 to 40 beats per minute. The inherent discharge of these pacemakers are not under vagal influence. They are thus not usually affected by exercise, emotion, respiration or atropine.

3. *The QRS configuration*

If the subsidiary pacemaker is situated in (*a*) the lower A-V node, i.e. below the block, or (*b*) in the bundle of His, the ectopic impulse activates the ventricles through normal or relatively normal pathways, and the QRS complex is normal, or near-normal, in shape (lead V1 in Fig. 168).

If the ectopic pacemaker is situated peripherally in the ventricular musculature, activation of the ventricles is bizarre, and the QRS complex is abnormal, being broad, notched, slurred and bizarre (Figs. 185, 186 and 187).

At times, two or more subsidiary pacemakers are in competition for the control of the ventricles. Thus, the ventricles may be temporarily under control of one pacemaker resulting in one form of QRS complex, followed by a change of QRS complex when control shifts to the other pacemaker. Stokes-Adams—syncopal—attacks (see below) not infrequently occur with a shift in pacemaker (Fig. 187).

VENTRICULAR ASYSTOLE

STOKES-ADAMS—SYNCOPAL—ATTACKS

A Stokes-Adams attack is a syncopal attack resulting from ventricular standstill or asystole, and occurs in third-degree A-V block when the subsidiary ectopic pacemaker fails to discharge (Figs. 185 and 187). It is most likely to occur under the following circumstances:

1.   During the *transition from incomplete (second-degree) to complete (third-degree) A-V block* when there may be some delay before a dormant or sluggish pacemaker is aroused and established.

Note: Complete A-V block that has been stable for a month or longer is uncommonly complicated by ventricular standstill and Stokes-Adams attack.

2.   When *two or more ectopic pacemakers are in competition*, a change or shift in pacemaker often heralds a Stokes-Adams attack—a period of asystole or ventricular standstill (Fig. 187).

Syncopal attacks may also be due to paroxysms of ventricular flutter or ventricular fibrillation. These attacks are also sometimes referred to as Stokes-Adams attacks.

'Giant' T wave inversion

When heart rhythm is complicated by ventricular asystole or paroxysmal ventricular flutter or fibrillation—giving rise to syncopal or Stokes-Adams attacks, the electrocardiogram frequently manifests with *very large, broad, bizarre and inverted T waves* (Fig. 184). The phenomenon is usually best seen in leads V2 to V4, and is partly an expression of marked prolongation of the Q–T interval: the Q–Tc may be increased to as much as 0.75 sec (Fig. 184). The manifestation has been termed 'Giant T wave inversion' (Jacobson &

Schrire, 1966[2]) and is very suggestive, indeed virtually pathognomonic, of a recent syncopal attack.

The definition of complete A-V block

There is at present no satisfactory definition of complete A-V block,
because most definitions do not take into account the effect of rate.
Even the definition of second-degree A-V block is not always
satisfactory, as rate is not usually taken into account. For example,
consider the case of an atrial flutter at a rate 300 beats per minute
which is associated with 2:1 A-V block. Is this true A-V block, or
merely the expression of the rapidly successive atrial flutter impulses
encountering the physiologic refractoriness of the A-V node? This is
almost certainly physiologic refractoriness and not a true A-V block.
The manifestation should, therefore, be referred to as 2:1 conduction
rather than 2:1 A-V block. At what supraventricular rate will the
advent of 2:1 conduction then connote true A-V block—the expression of an absolute increase in refractoriness? This has not yet
been established. The establishment of such a level may, indeed, be
impossible, for it may vary from case to case, and even at different
times in the same case. Furthermore, in cases of apparent complete
A-V dissociation, long recordings may reveal isolated capture-
conducted beats (Fig. 183).
    Complete A-V block could, then, possibly be defined as follows:
    *Complete A-V block is present when a fast or relatively fast
supraventricular rhythm is completely dissociated from a slow idionodal escape rhythm of less than 40 beats per minute or slow idioventricular rhythm of less than 35 beats per minute, and long recordings fail to
reveal any capture beats.*

High-grade A-V block

High-grade A-V block may be defined as intermittent block of two or
more consecutive supraventricular impulses. This definition, however, like the definition of complete A-V block unqualified by the
supraventricular rate (see above) is inadequate. Thus, the non-
conduction of two consecutive atrial flutter impulses may be physiological and may not reflect a true inherent increase in refractoriness.
At what rate then does the intermittent non-conduction of two or
more consecutive supraventricular impulses constitute a true high-
grade A-V block? The exact rate has not been established and may,
indeed, be impossible to establish. Nevertheless, an arbitrary supra-

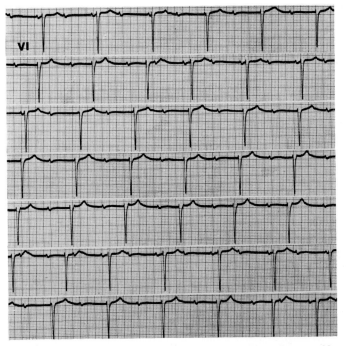

Fig. 183. The electrocardiogram (a continuous tracing of lead V1) shows: 1. *Normal sinus rhythm.* The P waves are normal. The intervals range from 0.75 sec to 0.82 sec, representing a sinus rate of 73 to 80 beats per minute. 2. *A-V dissociation between normal sinus rhythm and an idionodal escape rhythm.* This is evident from the complete dissociation (with three exceptions—see below) between the P waves and the normal QRS complexes. 3. *Idionodal escape rhythm.* This is evident from the normal QRS complexes. The R–R intervals of these complexes are constant at 1.49 sec, representing a rate of 40 beats per minute. 4. *Capture beats.* The A-V dissociation prevails throughout the tracing with three exceptions. Three QRS complexes are inscribed prematurely (R–R interval of 1.20 sec): fourth QRS complex in the second strip, third QRS complex in the sixth strip and the last QRS complex in the bottom strip. These QRS complexes are each preceded by a P wave at a P–R interval of 0.20 sec, reflecting a causal relationship. These QRS complexes are thus capture beats—the momentary conduction to, and capture of, the ventricles by the sinus impulse.

    Comment: 1. The A-V nodal origin of the escape rhythm is established by the fact that the QRS complexes of the escape beats are the same as the QRS complexes of the 3 conducted beats. 2. Conduction of the sinus impulse to the ventricles is only possible when the P wave occurs during a critical period after QRS complex, i.e. at a minimal R–P interval of 0.98 sec. All sinus impulses which occur at shorter R–P intervals are blocked. No conducted sinus impulses occur with P waves at longer R–P intervals, since the conduction of these relatively late sinus impulses are anticipated by the A-V nodal impulses. 3. *Note*: But for the 3 capture beats, this rhythm would be diagnosed as complete A-V block.

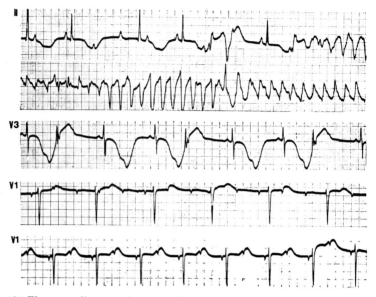

Fig. 184. Electrocardiograms showing: 1. Sinus rhythm complicated by high-grade A-V block. This is evident in the top strip. The second, fourth and seventh QRS complexes are preceded by P–R intervals of 0.14 sec and represent conducted sinus beats. The third and fourth sinus P waves are not conducted and are followed by A-V nodal escape beats. 2. Multiform ventricular flutter presenting as torsades de pointes. This is represented by the bizarre QRS complexes in Standard lead II which are recorded at a rate of 214 beats per minute. This patient experienced syncopal attacks which were due to the ventricular flutter. 3. 'Giant' T wave inversion and prolonged Q-Tc of 0.75 sec. This is best seen in lead V3. The manifestation is virtually pathognomonic of preceding episodes of unconsciousness. 3. Complete A-V block. This is evident in lead V1 (upper strip) and followed the administration of intravenous magnesium sulphate. 4. 2:1 A-V block. This occurred two hours later, and is depicted in lead V1 (lower strip).

ventricular rate of about 140 per minute would seem to be 'reasonable'. High-grade A-V block may thus tentatively be defined as the block of two or more consecutive supraventricular impulses at a rate of 140 per minute or less. See also section above on 'The Definition of Complete A-V Block'.

THE CAUSES OF COMPLETE A-V BLOCK

1. IDIOPATHIC SCLERODEGENERATIVE DISEASE: 'LENEGRE'S' DISEASE

Many cases of chronic complete A-V block are due to a sclero-

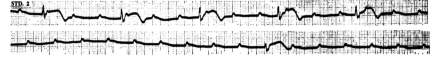

Fig. 185. Electrocardiogram (Standard lead II) showing: 1. Sinus rhythm complicated by *complete A-V block.* The P waves are unrelated—completely dissociated—from the bizarre QRS complexes of the idioventricular rhythm. The idioventricular rate is 30 beats per minute. 2. *A period of ventricular asystole* (which resulted in a Stokes-Adams attack). The fifth ventricular beat is followed by a period of asystole which is interrupted by a single ventricular beat.

degenerative process limited to the conducting system. The cause is unknown. Coronary artery disease does not play a significant role in its pathogenesis. Lenegre (1958)[3] was the first to describe it.

2. CORONARY ARTERY DISEASE

Coronary artery disease, particularly acute anterior wall myocardial infarction, may cause complete A-V block. The association with acute anterior wall myocardial infarction usually carries a very adverse prognosis. Indeed, the occurrence of any form of A-V block as a complication of acute myocardial infarction worsens the prognosis. The higher the degree of block, the worse the prognosis (Cohen and associates, 1958[1]).

3. FIBROCALCAREOUS ENCROACHMENT: 'LEV'S' DISEASE

Complete A-V block may result from the extension of a fibrocalcareous process which may involve the aortic valve (aortic stenosis), the pars membranacea, the mitral annulus, and the summit of the interventricular septum. Encroachment of the disease process upon the neighbouring conducting system may cause any degree of A-V block. The condition usually occurs in elderly people and has received emphasis by Lev (1964).[4]

4. INTRACARDIAC SURGERY

Surgery in the vicinity of the conducting system may cause complete A-V block either by direct severance of the conducting system, or as a result of oedema and pressure upon the conducting system.

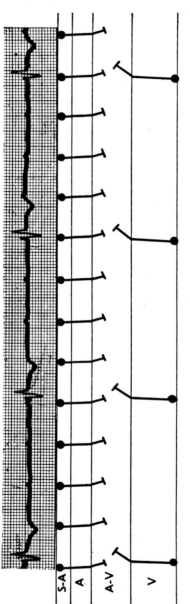

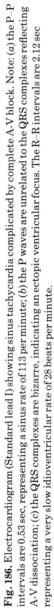

Fig. 186. Electrocardiogram (Standard lead I) showing sinus tachycardia complicated by complete A-V block. Note: (*a*) the P–P intervals are 0.53 sec, representing a sinus rate of 113 per minute; (*b*) the P waves are unrelated to the QRS complexes reflecting A-V dissociation; (*c*) the QRS complexes are bizarre, indicating an ectopic ventricular focus. The R–R intervals are 2.12 sec representing a very slow idioventricular rate of 28 beats per minute.

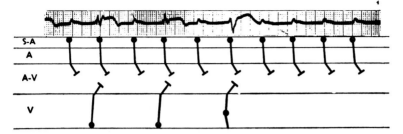

Fig. 187. Electrocardiogram (Standard lead II) showing sinus rhythm complicated by complete A-V block. Note (*a*) the P waves are unrelated to the QRS complexes; (*b*) the QRS complexes are bizarre indicating an ectopic ventricular origin; (*c*) the third QRS complex differs from the other two indicating a change in ventricular focus; this change precipitates ventricular standstill or asystole leading to a Stokes-Adams attack.

5. DIGITALIS INTOXICATION

Digitalis intoxication may rarely cause complete A-V block. When this occurs, there is usually a concomitant underlying pathology such as degenerative or coronary artery disease. In other words, digitalis intoxication rarely causes third-degree A-V block unless there is some associated disease; whereas it readily causes first- or second-degree A-V block.

6. TUMOURS, PARASITIC INFESTATIONS, PYOGENIC AND GRANULOMATOUS INFECTIONS

These diseases may involve the conducting system and cause complete A-V block. They are, however, very rare causes of complete A-V block and may be regarded as clinical curiosities. In Central and South America, however, Chaga's disease is probably the commonest cause of A-V block.

7. CONGENITAL HEART DISEASE

Complete A-V block is not infrequently associated with congenital heart disease such as corrected transposition of the great vessels, ventricular septal defect and ostium primum type of atrial septal defect.

8. CONGENITAL A-V BLOCK

Complete A-V block may occur as an isolated congenital anomaly. It has the following electrocardiographic features:

A. The block is nearly always within the A-V node and the subsidiary pacemaker is situated distal to the block within the lower part of the A-V node or the bundle of His. *The QRS complexes are therefore normal.*

B. The idionodal rate is usually in the rate-range of 55 to 65 beats per minute, i.e. in a slightly higher rate-range than that usually associated with acquired complete A-V block.

C. The ventricular rate tends to fluctuate slightly with emotion and exercise, i.e. it appears to be under some autonomic influence and is, therefore, less stable than the rhythm usually associated with the acquired forms of complete A-V block.

D. Syncopal attacks are very rare.

Note. acute rheumatic carditis may be associated with first- or second-degree A-V block, but is not associated with third-degree or complete A-V block.

REFERENCES

1 Cohen D. B., Doctor L. & Pick A. (1958) The significance of atrioventricular block complicating acute myocardial infarction. *Amer. Heart J.* **55,** 215.

2 Jacobson D. & Schrire V. (1966) Giant T-wave inversion. *Brit. Heart J.* **28,** 768.

3 Lenegre J. (1958) *Contribution a l'Etude des Blocs de Branche.* Paris: J. B. Ballière et Fils.

4 Lev M. (1964) Anatomic basis of atrioventricular block. *Amer. J. Med.* **37,** 742.

Chapter 19
Reciprocal Rhythm

Reciprocal rhythm refers to a conduction sequence wherein an impulse arises in the S-A node, the atria, the A-V node or the ventricles, and during, or after, its conduction through the A-V node, enters another A-V junctional pathway or by-pass which enables it to return to and activate the atria or the ventricles once again (Fig. 188). In other words, the atria or the ventricles are activated two or more times by the *same* impulse, and this can only occur if there are at least two pathways within the A-V junction.

BASIC PREDISPOSING CONDITIONS

The essential predisposing conditions to reciprocal rhythm are:
1.   The presence of an additional A-V pathway—a by-pass.
2.   The presence of *differential refractoriness* within the two A-V pathways: *a functional unidirectional block in the reciprocal pathway*.
3.   A relatively prolonged reciprocal time when a common A-V nodal pathway is used in the reciprocal circuit (see section below on 'An additional intranodal pathway').

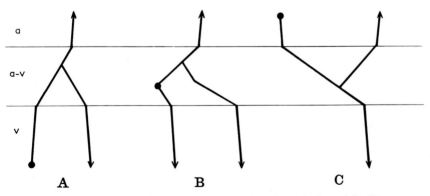

Fig. 188. Diagrams illustrating: (A) reciprocal rhythm of ventricular origin, (B) reciprocal rhythm of A-V nodal origin and (C) reciprocal rhythm of atrial origin. The by-pass is situated within the A-V node.

1. The additional A-V pathway: the A-V by-pass

Reciprocal rhythm can only occur if there are at least two separate pathways within the A-V junction. There are four potential anatomical structures which could constitute the necessary A-V by-pass, and thereby form the necessary substrate for reciprocal rhythm (Fig. 189). These are:

(*a*) *The bundle of Kent*: This is a thin filamentous structure, congenital in origin, which may be situated ectopically anywhere along the A-V ring—the fibrous structure separating the atria from the ventricles. It is completely separate from the A-V node and bundle of His (Figs. 189 and 194. See also Chapter 21).

(*b*) *A Mahaim Fibre*: This is a thin filamentous structure, congenital in origin which arises in the A-V node or the bundle of His,

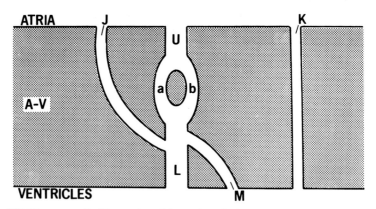

Fig. 189. Diagrammatic illustration of the various A-V junctional pathways which constitute the anatomical substrate for reciprocal rhythm. J = James bypass. K = Kent bundle. M = Mahaim fibre. a and b = two intranodal pathways. U = upper common pathway. L = lower common pathway.

and, so-to-speak, ends 'blindly' within the ventricular myocardium (Figs. 189 and 194).

(*c*) *The James By-Pass*: This is a conduction pathway which, in effect, extends from the atria by-passing the main body of the A-V node to insert distally into the A-V node (Figs. 189, 194 and 205).

(*d*) *An additional intranodal pathway*: An additional intranodal pathway is usually situated in the middle of the A-V node. The two pathways communicate with each other in both the upper and lower parts of the A-V node to form both upper and lower common pathways (Figs. 189 and 194).

2. The reciprocal pathway and unidirectional block

The essential prerequisite to the initiation of any reciprocal rhythm is unequal refractoriness or responsiveness of the two A-V nodal pathways. This condition is necessary so that an impulse arising, for example, in the ventricles, will enter one pathway only and then return in the opposite direction through the other pathway. If the two pathways were equally responsive the impulse would enter both pathways simultaneously and then proceed in the same direction through both pathways. Retrograde return through either pathway would then become impossible and a reciprocal mechanism would, thereby, be obviated. This is, indeed, the case in the classic form of Wolff-Parksinon-White conduction when the sinus impulse enters two A-V junctional pathways simultaneously; conduction proceeds anterogradely through both pathways, and subsequent intraventricular conduction results in the typical Wolff-Parkinson-White fusion complexes. When, however, the refractory periods of the two pathways become unequal, the atrial impulse enters one pathway only, returns retrogradely through the other pathway and, thereby, initiates reciprocal rhythm. Transient functional unidirectional block must, therefore, exist in one of the conduction pathways to enable the development of a reciprocal mechanism.

3. An adequate or relatively prolonged reciprocal time when a common pathway is used

An adequate—relatively prolonged—time must elapse for the reciprocal impulse to effect its circuit when such circuit includes an upper and/or a lower common A-V nodal pathway. This is necessary, in reciprocal rhythm of atrial origin, to allow the atria and/or an upper common pathway sufficient time for recovery following their initial activation, so that they can respond to the reciprocal impulse once again. A prolonged reciprocal time may also be necessary, in the case of reciprocal rhythm of A-V nodal or ventricular origin, to allow for the recovery of a lower common pathway and/or the ventricles.

ELECTROCARDIOGRAPHIC MANIFESTATIONS

Reciprocal rhythm may occur with impulses of atrial, A-V nodal or ventricular origin.

1. Reciprocal rhythm with an impulse of atrial origin

Basic mechanism. In reciprocal rhythm of atrial origin, a supraventricular impulse—most commonly a sinus impulse—activates the atria and is then conducted anterogradely through the A-V node to activate the ventricles. Reciprocal return to the atria may then occur within the A-V node, i.e. during its passage through the A-V node the impulse also enters another intranodal pathway and is, thereby, conducted retrogradely through this pathway to activate the atria once again (Fig. 190). The impulse may, however, only begin its return to the atria once it has reached the ventricles. The return would then be effected by either: (*a*) a Mahaim fibre in which case it still has to traverse an upper common pathway (illustrated in Diagrams C and G of Fig. 194), or (*b*) a Kent bundle (illustrated in Diagrams D and H of Fig. 194).

ELECTROCARDIOGRAPHIC MANIFESTATIONS

Reciprocal rhythm of atrial origin is reflected by a basic P-QRS-P′ sequence.

The initial P wave is the result of normal activation by the sinus impulse. The QRS complex is the result of normal anterograde A-V conduction to the ventricles.

The P′ deflection—also known as an *atrial echo*—is the result of reciprocal retrograde activation of the atria (Fig. 190). In cases of intranodal re-entry or retrograde return through a Mahaim fibre, the P–R interval of the basic reciprocal sequence is usually prolonged, reflecting a prolonged anterograde conduction time. This is necessary to effect the necessary prolonged re-entry time, so that the common upper pathway has sufficient recovery time and is able to

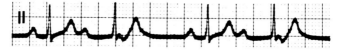

Fig. 190. Electrocardiogram (Standard lead II) showing a basic sinus rhythm conducted with a Wenckebach-like sequence. The first sinus impulse of the sequence is conducted with a P–R interval of 0.24 sec. The second P–R interval is further prolonged to 0·40 sec. This long P–R interval is followed by an inverted P′ wave which is superimposed upon and deforms the ensuing S-T segment. This P′ wave is always selectively linked to a prolonged P–R interval and reflects an atrial echo: the reciprocal return of a sinus impulse through an additional intranodal pathway and an upper common pathway.

(*Courtesy of Dr Hernandes Pieretti*)

respond to the re-entering impulse. Thus, it is commonly observed that the reciprocal beat—the 'retrograde' or P′ deflection in any one tracing—only occurs after a prolonged P–R interval; whereas no such P′ deflections follow relatively short P–R intervals. In other words, the reciprocal P′ deflections are selectively linked to preceding P–R intervals (Fig. 190).

2. Reciprocal rhythm with an impulse of A-V nodal origin

Basic mechanism. In reciprocal rhythm of A-V nodal origin, an impulse arising in the A-V node is conducted in two directions:

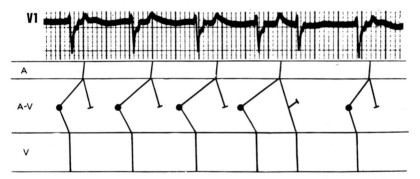

Fig. 191. The electrocardiogram (lead V1) shows: 1. *Idionodal tachycardia.* The QRS complexes resemble the QRS complexes of conducted sinus impulses (observed at other times and not illustrated). This indicates a supraventricular origin. The QRS complexes are related to succeeding P′ waves. These P′ waves may be seen superimposed upon S-T segments and T waves. The R–R intervals of the first three cycles measures 0.54 sec, reflecting a rate of 110 beats per minute. 2. *Retrograde Wenckebach conduction.* There is a progressive increase in the R–P intervals: 0.13 sec, 0.16 sec, 0.18 sec and 0.19 sec, reflecting a retrograde Wenckebach conduction sequence. 3. *A reciprocal sequence.* The idionodal beat with the longest R–P interval is associated with a succeeding prematurely inscribed QRS complex of the same configuration as that recorded by the A-V nodal beats. The prematurity of this QRS complex results in an R–R interval of 0.37 sec. This prematurely inscribed QRS complex was repeatedly observed and was always associated with the longest R–P′ intervals. Furthermore, it always resulted in an R–R interval of 0.37 sec. This indicates a causal relationship of the premature QRS complex to the preceding A-V nodal beat. The fact that this premature QRS complex is only associated with an A-V nodal beat having a long R–P′ interval indicates the presence of a reciprocal mechanism. The long retrograde conduction time facilitates the recovery of a lower common A-V nodal pathway, and thus enables the completion of the reciprocal circuit (as diagrammed). A second reciprocal circuit is blocked and this facilitates the recovery of the retrograde pathway so that the ensuing A-V nodal beat is conducted with a relatively short R–P′ interval (0.13 sec) once again.

anterogradely to the ventricles and retrogradely to the atria. The retrogradely conducted impulse, during its passage through the A-V node may also enter another A-V intranodal pathway which enables it to return anterogradely to, and activate, the ventricles once again (Diagram B of Fig. 188).

ELECTROCARDIOGRAPHIC MANIFESTATIONS

Reciprocal rhythm with impulses of A-V nodal origin is classically reflected by a QRS-P'-QRS sequence or 'sandwich' (Fig. 191). The initial QRS complex is the result of normal anterograde conduction of the A-V nodal impulse to, and activation of, the ventricles. The P' deflection is the result of retrograde activation of the atria. The second QRS complex is the result of reciprocal activation of ventricles, and may be aberrantly conducted.

3. Reciprocal rhythm with an impulse of ventricular origin

Basic mechanism. In reciprocal rhythm of ventricular origin, a ventricular impulse activates the ventricles, and is then conducted retrogradely through the A-V node to activate the atria.

Reciprocal return to the ventricles may occur within the A-V node (Diagram A of Fig. 188) or, after having reached the atria through a Kent bundle or a James by-pass, in which case it would have to traverse a lower common pathway. The reactivation of the ventricles constitutes a reciprocal beat and is also known as a *return extrasystole*.

ELECTROCARDIOGRAPHIC MANIFESTATIONS

Reciprocal rhythm of ventricular origin is reflected by a QRS-P'-QRS sequence (Fig. 192).

The initial QRS complex is the result of ventricular activation by an extrasystolic ventricular impulse and is, therefore, abnormal and bizarre.

The P' deflection is the result of retrograde activation of the atria. The second QRS complex of the reciprocal sequence is the result of reciprocal activation of the ventricles by the returning impulse. The returning impulse usually follows normal intraventricular conduction pathways and the resulting QRS complex can, therefore, be completely normal in configuration. However, because of its relative prematurity, the returning impulse may be conducted with aber-

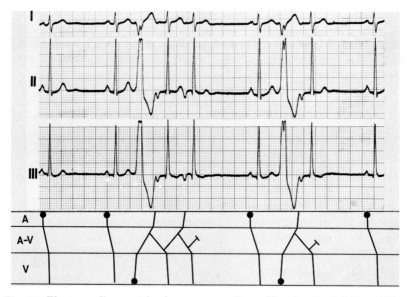

Fig. 192. Electrocardiogram (simultaneous recordings of Standard leads I, II and III) shows the following features: 1. *Sinus tachycardia*. This is reflected by the first 2 beats. The P–P interval measures 1.13 sec representing a rate of 53 per minute. 2. *A ventricular extrasystole initiating reciprocal rhythm*. The bizarre and premature QRS complex which occurs after the second conducted beat represents a ventricular extrasystole. This is associated with retrograde conduction to the atria as reflected by the ensuing inverted P′ wave. This is followed by a reciprocal return to the ventricles resulting in a reciprocal beat having a normal QRS configuration. This is followed by a further retrograde return to the atria as evidenced by the ensuing retrograde inverted P′ wave, and another reciprocal beat. Retrograde conduction following this beat is blocked. This is followed by another sinus beat, a ventricular extrasystole and a further reciprocal beat.

ration which will modify the QRS configuration. Whether the returning impulse is conducted normally or with phasic aberrant ventricular conduction, the resulting QRS complex is markedly different from the initial QRS complex.

RECIPROCATING RHYTHM: RECIPROCATING TACHYCARDIA

The returning impulse, no matter which reciprocal pathway is used and irrespectively of its origin, may re-enter the original A-V pathway once again and, thereby, complete two or more further circuits. This results in a reciprocating rhythm—a reciprocating tachycardia. This is considered further in Chapter 20.

Chapter 20
The Supraventricular Tachycardias

A plethora of publications during the past decade has necessitated a re-appraisal of the whole concept of supraventricular tachycardia. The simplified view, previously held, that the term is used for atrial and A-V nodal tachycardia where the precise origin cannot be established, is an oversimplification which is no longer tenable. Many supraventricular tachycardias which were previously thought to be an expression of enhanced automaticity, are now known to be reciprocating mechanisms which may be associated with various reciprocal pathways (see Chapter 19).

Many forms of supraventricular tachycardia have consequently been recognized and their properties and mechanisms identified on the basis of new electrophysiological techniques, as well as analysis of the conventional clinical electrocardiogram. It has thus become necessary, when appraising the concept of supraventricular tachycardia, to determine not only the site of impulse of origin, but also whether the tachycardia is an expression of enhanced automaticity or a reciprocating mechanism; and in the case of a reciprocating mechanism, the anatomical circuit involved. Some of these factors are briefly considered below.

THE BASIC FORMS OF SUPRAVENTRICULAR TACHYCARDIA

Supraventricular tachycardia may be due to enhanced focal automaticity or a reciprocating mechanism. The basic differentiation between these two forms is based on the following criteria:

1. The significance of second degree A-V block

One of the most important criteria for separating supraventricular tachycardia due to focal automaticity from reciprocating junctional tachycardia is the presence of second degree A-V block. Reciprocating A-V junctional tachycardia can only exist with 1:1 conduction (Figs. 193 and 206) since a continuous, reciprocating, circuitous

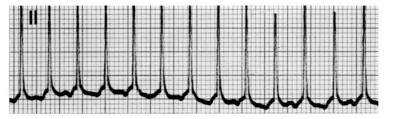

Fig. 193. The electrocardiogram (Standard II) reflects a tachycardia with narrow QRS complexes representing a supraventricular origin. The R–R intervals measure 0.26 sec representing a rate of 231 per minute. Each QRS complex is followed by an inverted P′ wave reflecting 1:1 conduction with probable retrograde conduction. This manifestation almost certainly reflects a supraventricular reciprocating tachycardia.

process must be terminated by any event which interrupts the circuit. Thus, when second-degree A-V block complicates a supraventricular tachycardia, the diagnosis of a reciprocating mechanism involving a Kent bundle or Mahaim fibre can be definitely ruled out. Even a single episode of A-V block occurring anywhere within the reciprocal circuit must terminate the tachycardia. Consequently, atrial tachycardia with established second- or third-degree A-V block usually reflects the mechanism of enhanced focal automaticity.

Similarly, an A-V junctional tachycardia with: (*a*) second-degree retrograde or anterograde A-V block, or (*b*) persistent A-V dissociation from an atrial rhythm will rule out a reciprocating mechanism, especially one involving Kent bundle conduction.

2. The P wave morphology

The P wave morphology may at times suggest the mechanism present but is not diagnostic with present-day criteria. For example, negative P′ waves in Standard lead I, and in leads V5 and V6 may suggest a reciprocating mechanism involving a left-sided Kent bundle. This is because retrograde conduction through such a bundle will result in an atrial activation front which is directed upwards and to the right; and which would consequently be directed away from the positive poles of Standard lead I and leads V5 and V6.

3. The P:QRS relationship

The absence of visible P waves strongly suggests an intranodal reciprocating tachycardia. This is because of simultaneous, or almost simultaneous, atrial and ventricular activation so that the P′ wave is hidden within the QRS complex. With tachycardia due to focal automaticity the P′ wave is usually well clear of the QRS complex. Furthermore, if the P′ wave of the first—initiating—premature atrial depolarization is the same as the ensuing P′ waves of the tachycardia, focal automaticity is the likely mechanism.

A critical initial prolongation of A-V conduction time—as reflected by a prolonged P–R interval—is frequently associated with, and is necessary for, some forms of reciprocating tachycardia. No such prolongation is necessary for the initiation of a focal tachycardia.

4. The effect of electric stimulation

A critically timed intracardiac electric stimulus, or paired electric stimuli, will almost invariably terminate a reciprocating tachycardia. It may also terminate a focal tachycardia, but the effect is uncertain and, therefore, not predictable.

ELECTROCARDIOGRAPHIC POINTERS TO THE PRESENCE OF RECIPROCATING TACHYCARDIA

The following electrocardiographic features are pointers to the presence of a reciprocating mechanism in a tachycardia.

1.   Tachycardia which occurs without second-degree A-V block, i.e. with a persistent 1:1 relationship of atrial to ventricular depolarization is a strong pointer to the presence of a reciprocal mechanism. (Fig. 193).

2.   Physiological or pharmacological vagotonic procedures, or the administration of other antiarrhythmic agents, do not induce second-degree A-V block, or terminate the tachycardia without preliminary disturbance of the 1:1 relationship.

3.   When a tachycardia presents with bizarre QRS complexes, a 1:1 relationship of atrial to ventricular depolarization will also favour a reciprocating tachycardia. Conversely, when a tachycardia presents with bizarre QRS complexes, the association of second-degree retrograde A-V block effectively rules out a reciprocal mechanism and indicates the presence of ventricular tachycardia.

4.   A rate less than 120 beats per minute is quite exceptional in reciprocating tachycardia.

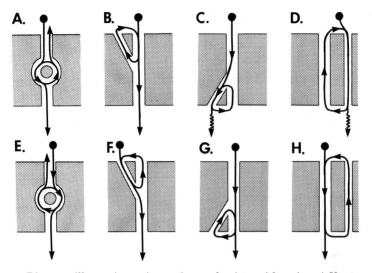

Fig. 194. Diagrams illustrating reciprocating mechanisms with various A-V junctional anatomical pathways. Diagrams A and E represent intranodal reciprocation. Diagrams B and F represent reciprocation through a James by-pass. Diagrams C and G represent reciprocation through a Mahaim fibre. Diagrams D and H represent reciprocation through a Kent bundle (see text).

COMMENTS

1.   The precise origin of the initiating impulse may be evident when the beginning of the tachycardia is recorded, but may be difficult to determine during the course of the actual tachycardia. Furthermore, a reciprocating tachycardia, once initiated by a specific impulse origin, may be interrupted by, and then continued by, an impulse of different origin. For example, a reciprocating tachycardia precipitated by a sinus impulse can be interrupted by an ectopic ventricular impulse or a single electric ventricular stimulus. The interruption may terminate the tachycardia, or may re-set the cycle and continue the tachycardia.

2.   Conduction through an anatomical reciprocal circuit may occur potentially in either direction, i.e. it may be 'clockwise' or 'counter-clockwise'. Thus, an A-V pathway forming part of the circuit may potentially transmit the impulse in either direction (compare Diagrams A, B, C and D with Diagrams E, F, G and H in Fig. 194). However, the refractory state of the A-V junctional pathways is usually such that the refractory period of the accessory pathway to anterograde conduction is longer than that of the A-V node itself.

Thus, anterograde—atrioventricular—conduction is nearly always through the A-V nodal-His-Purkinje system, with retrograde—ventriculoatrial—conduction through the accessory pathway. On rare occasions, the reciprocating circuit may be associated with anterograde conduction through the accessory pathway and retrograde conduction through the A-V node. This has also been termed 'antidromic reciprocating tachycardia'.

Chapter 21
The Wolff-Parkinson-White
and Related Syndromes

The Wolff-Parkinson-White (W-P-W) syndrome (1930)[4] is an electro-cardiographic syndrome resulting from concomitant normal and anomalous conduction of the atrial impulse to the ventricles. It has the following characteristics (Figs. 195, 197, 200, 201 and 202).

1.   **A shortened P–R interval.**
2.   **A widened QRS complex.**
3.   A slurred and thickened proximal limb of the QRS complex—designated the **delta wave.**
4.   A normal or relatively normal narrow terminal deflection of the QRS complex.
5.   Secondary S-T segment and T wave changes.

The P–R interval is shortened by as much as the QRS complex is widened, as though the proximal limb of the QRS complex has been 'pulled towards' the P wave (Fig. 195).

MECHANISM

The abnormality is due to the presence of an *anomalous pathway*—an additional A-V pathway or by-pass—probably congenital in origin, between the atria and ventricles (Figs. 196, 198 and 199). The anomalous pathway may be situated anywhere along the A-V ring, and is known as the bundle of Kent.

The atrial impulse travels down *both* the normal and anomalous pathways concomitantly (Figs. 196A, 198 and 199A) but is conducted at a faster rate down the anomalous pathway. It thus reaches the ventricles earlier than the normally conducted impulse and results in the early inscription of the QRS complex—hence the shortened P–R interval. Once this impulse reaches the ventricles, however, further onward or caudal transmission is not through specialized conducting tissue but through ordinary myocardium which is a poor conducting medium. Further conduction is, therefore, slower than normal, producing the bizarre, slurred, delta wave. The early bizarre acti-vation of part of the ventricular myocardium is known as pre-

233

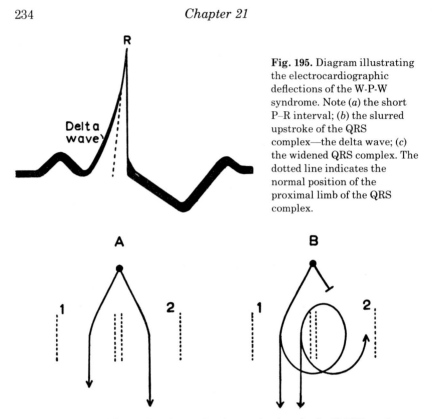

Fig. 195. Diagram illustrating the electrocardiographic deflections of the W-P-W syndrome. Note (*a*) the short P–R interval; (*b*) the slurred upstroke of the QRS complex—the delta wave; (*c*) the widened QRS complex. The dotted line indicates the normal position of the proximal limb of the QRS complex.

Fig. 196. Diagrams illustrating the conduction mechanisms in the W-P-W syndrome. (1) Normal pathway, i.e. the A-V node. (2) Anomalous pathway. (A) illustrates the conduction mechanism that inscribes the typical W-P-W fusion complex, i.e. the atrial impulse is conducted through both pathways concomitantly but at a faster rate through the anomalous pathway. (B) illustrates conduction during paroxysmal tachycardia, viz. anterograde conduction through the normal pathway and retrograde conduction through the anomalous pathway.

excitation; and the part so activated is known as the pre-excitation area.

Conduction through the A-V node proceeds normally but at a slower rate than through the anomalous pathway. Once it reaches the ventricles, however, further transmission is through normal, quick conducting, specialized tissue, viz. the bundle of His, the bundle branches and Purkinje network. Consequently, the impulse conducted through the A-V node eventually 'overtakes' the impulse conducted through the anomalous pathway and records the rest of the QRS complex which is, therefore, normal, or near normal (Fig. 198). The potential modifications of the narrow terminal QRS deflection are considered below. Thus the typical complex of the W-P-W syndrome is a form of **fusion complex:** the initial part—the delta wave—is recorded by that part of the sinus impulse conducted through the anomalous pathway; and the normal part of the QRS complex is recorded by that part of the sinus impulse conducted through the A-V node.

THE TYPE A AND TYPE B W-P-W SYNDROME

The W-P-W syndrome may be classified into two types, based on the direction of the dominant QRS deflection in the right precordial leads: leads V1 and V2 (Rosenbaum and associates, 1945[1]).

THE TYPE A W-P-W SYNDROME

The Type A W-P-W syndrome is characterized by a dominantly upright QRS deflection in the right precordial leads, resulting in tall R waves in leads V1 and V2 (Fig. 200).

　　The by-pass in the Type A W-P-W syndrome is usually situated on the left, i.e. the pre-excitation area is usually the left ventricle.

THE TYPE B W-P-W SYNDROME

The Type B W-P-W syndrome is characterized by a dominantly negative QRS deflection in the right precordial leads (Fig. 197).

　　When the Type B W-P-W syndrome is associated with cyanotic congenital heart disease, it is said to be pathognomonic of Ebstein's Anomaly (Sodi-Pallares & Calder, 1956[3]).

　　The by-pass in the Type B W-P-W syndrome is usually situated on the right, i.e. the pre-excitation area is usually in the right ventricle.

POTENTIAL MODIFICATION OF THE TERMINAL QRS DEFLECTION

Although the terminal part of the QRS deflection is narrow and thus represents relatively normal ventricular activation it may, nevertheless, still be modified. The modifications are best seen when the W-P-W syndrome is intermittent and can thus be compared with normal uncomplicated intraventricular conduction. The modifications may take two forms:

1.　An increase in the amplitude of the terminal deflection (Fig. 203).

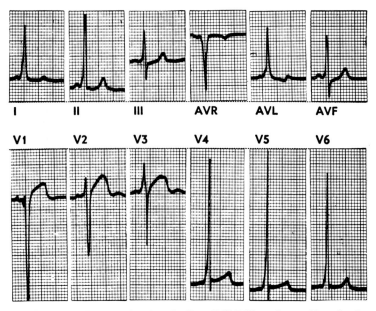

I   II   III   AVR   AVL   AVF

V1   V2   V3   V4   V5   V6

Fig. 197. Electrocardiogram showing the Type B W-P-W syndrome. Note the short P–R interval, delta wave, and widened QRS complex—well seen in most leads.

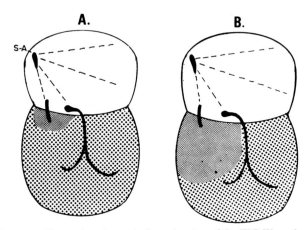

Fig. 198. Diagrams illustrating the typical conduction of the W-P-W syndrome. The darker shading reflects the pre-excitation area: the contribution to ventricular activation by the impulse conducted through the by-pass. Pre-excitation is greater in Diagram B than in Diagram A.

2.   An axis deviation of the terminal part of the QRS deflection (Fig. 203).

There may be either right or left axis deviation. Such deviation is more likely to occur with the Type A Wolf-Parkinson-White syndrome (Schamroth, 1975[2]).

THE SIGNIFICANCE OF THE W-P-W SYNDROME

The W-P-W syndrome has two important implications:
1.   Individuals with the W-P-W syndrome are prone to attacks of **supraventricular tachyarrhythmias:**
    A.   Reciprocating tachycardia.
    B.   Paroxysmal atrial flutter or paroxysmal atrial fibrillation.
2.   The W-P-W syndrome may mimic other electrocardiographic manifestations and lead to erroneous diagnosis.

1. THE SUPRAVENTRICULAR TACHYARRHYTHMIAS

A. *Reciprocating tachycardia*

Anterograde conduction through the anomalous pathway may at times be blocked. The sinus impulse may then travel anterogradely through the normal pathway only but is able to return retrogradely through the anomalous pathway—retrograde Kent bundle conduction (Figs. 196B and 199B). It may then travel anterogradely through the normal A-V nodal once again. And if this mechanism continues, a *circus movement* is established between the normal and anomalous A-V pathways resulting in a tachycardia. This is a form of reciprocal rhythm, and the resulting tachycardia is known as a reciprocating tachycardia.

Since anterograde conduction during the tachycardia usually occurs through the normal A-V nodal pathway only, no delta wave is inscribed. Thus, the typical complex of the W-P-W syndrome disappears during the tachycardia (Fig 202). Furthermore, since the mechanism is a circus movement, it is clear that the tachycardia cannot be complicated by second-degree A-V block; any block of the circus movement would immediately terminate the tachycardia.

Note. Atrial tachycardias of focal origin are usually associated with second-degree A-V block when the rate exceeds 200 beats per minute. The reciprocating tachycardia of the W-P-W syndrome, however, can be conducted without block even when the rate exceeds 200 beats per minute (Fig. 202, lower strip).

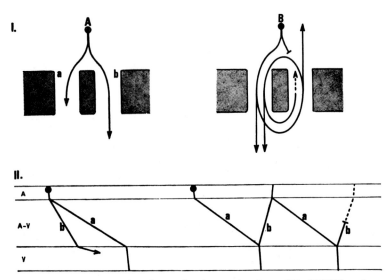

Fig. 199. Diagrams illustrating the conduction mechanisms of the W-P-W syndrome: (a) represents the normal pathway; (b) represents the anomalous pathway.

Diagram A illustrates the conduction mechanism responsible for the typical W-P-W pattern, i.e. the sinus impulse is conducted through both pathways concomitantly but at a faster rate through the anomalous pathway. Diagram B illustrates the conduction mechanism responsible for the reciprocating—paroxysmal—tachycardia, i.e. anterograde conduction through the normal pathway and retrograde conduction through the anomalous pathway: retrograde Kent bundle conduction.

B. *Paroxysmal atrial flutter or fibrillation*

The initiation of atrial fibrillation or atrial flutter in the W-P-W syndrome is brought about by the basic reciprocal mechanism facilitated by the anomalous by-pass. The by-pass permits the rapid and early return of the supraventricular impulse to the atria; and the returning impulse may, as a result, reach the atria at the end of their refractory period—during their early simple out-of-phase state or vulnerable phase. Atrial fibrillation or flutter may, therefore, be precipitated. Since a large atrial mass (as found in acquired heart disease) is necessary to maintain fibrillation or flutter, the fibrillation or flutter of the W-P-W syndrome is rarely maintained for long periods and is consequently paroxysmal in nature.

2. CONDITIONS SIMULATED BY THE W-P-W SYNDROME

The W-P-W syndrome may simulate the following conditions:

A. *Myocardial infarction*

A negative-delta wave in Standard lead I and lead AVL may simulate anterolateral wall myocardial infarction (Fig. 200). A negative delta wave in Standard lead III and lead AVF may simulate inferior wall myocardial infarction (Fig. 201). The tall R waves in the right

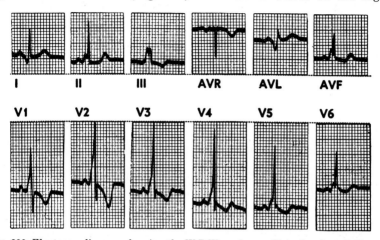

Fig. 200. Electrocardiogram showing the W-P-W syndrome. Note the short P–R interval, delta wave and widened QRS complex—well seen in most leads. The delta wave is negative in Standard lead I and lead AVL and may be mistaken for the pathological Q wave of an anterolateral myocardial infarction.

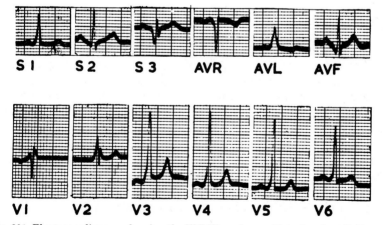

Fig. 201. Electrocardiogram showing the W-P-W syndrome. Note the short P–R interval, delta wave and widened QRS complex—well seen in most leads. The delta wave is negative in Standard lead III and AVF and may be mistaken for the pathological Q wave of inferior myocardial infarction.

A

B

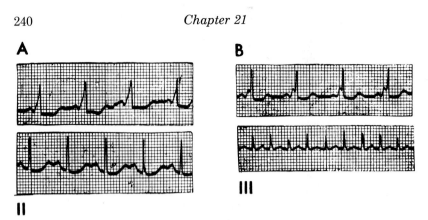

II

III

Fig. 202. Electrocardiograms A and B are from different patients with the W-P-W syndrome. The upper strips are recorded during slow rates and show the typical QRS pattern, viz. delta wave, widened QRS complex and short P–R interval. The lower strips were recorded from the same patients using the same leads and show the disappearance of the typical QRS pattern during paroxysmal tachycardia.

precordial leads in the Type A W-P-W syndrome may simulate true posterior wall infarction.

B. *Right ventricular hypertrophy*

The tall R waves in the right precordial leads in the Type A W-P-W syndrome may simulate right ventricular hypertrophy (Fig. 200).

C. *Bundle branch block*

The combination of a prominent delta wave and QRS complex may result in the appearance of a 'notched' QRS complex which may simulate bundle branch block (e.g. leads V1 and V2 in Fig. 201).

D. *Simulated primary myocardial disease*

Secondary S-T segment and T wave changes—S-T segment depression, horizontality, and T wave inversion—may be associated with the abnormal intraventricular depolarization of the W-P-W syndrome. These secondary S-T segment and T wave changes may be mistaken for the primary S-T segment and T wave changes of myocardial disease (e.g. leads V1 to V6 in Fig. 200).

MAHAIM FIBRE PRE-EXCITATION

A Mahaim fibre is a fibre which is congenital in origin and which

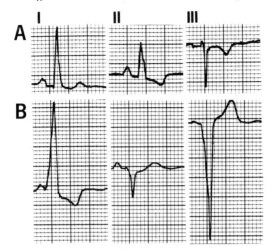

Fig. 203. Electrocardiograms recorded from the same patient showing: (A) Normal intraventricular conduction; (B) W-P-W conduction. Note the development of left axis deviation and increased QRS amplitude with pre-excitation.

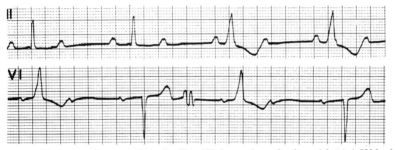

Fig. 204. Electrocardiograms: Standard lead II shows sinus rhythm with 2:1 A-V block, the conducted beat having a prolonged P–R interval. The third and fourth beats reflect pre-excitation with a relatively normal P–R interval, thereby indicating Mahaim fibre conduction. Lead V1 shows sinus rhythm with 2:1 A-V block, the first and third conducted beats exhibiting the pre-excitation and normal P–R interval of Mahaim fibre conduction.

arises distally in the A-V node and ends 'blindly' so-to-speak in the ventricular myocardium (Fig. 189). A sinus impulse may consequently be conducted through the A-V node and then through a Mahaim fibre to pre-excite the ventricles. This, too, will result in a delta wave. Unlike Kent bundle pre-excitation, however, the sinus impulse must be conducted through the main region of physiological delay within the A-V node before onward conduction occurs through both the Mahaim fibre and the His bundle. Thus Mahaim fibre pre-excitation has the same features of the Wolff-Parkinson-White syndrome but is associated with a normal P–R interval (Fig. 204).

THE LOWN-GANONG-LEVINE SYNDROME: SYNDROME OF SHORT P–R INTERVAL AND NORMAL QRS COMPLEX

The Lown-Ganong-Levine (L.G.L.) syndrome is characterized by a normal P wave, a short P–R interval, and a normal QRS complex (Fig. 206). Individuals with this syndrome are also prone to attacks of paroxysmal tachycardia.

   This syndrome is due to a James by-pass, a pathway which arises in the atria and by-passes the main region of conduction delay within the A-V node to end distally in the A-V node or the bundle of His (Fig. 205). Thus, unlike the anomalous pathway of a W.P.W. syndrome, the James by-pass does not end in, or activate, the myocardium directly; hence the absence of bizarre anomalous activation as reflected by the delta wave. The absence of anomalous ventricular activation indicates that the by-pass joins the bundle of His or lower part of the A-V node directly (Fig. 205). The sinus impulse is thus able to short-circuit the major conduction impediment of the A-V node, resulting in earlier activation of the ventricles as reflected by a short P–R interval. Its further onward or intraventricular conduction can still occur through the normal specialized conducting system (bundle of His and the bundle branches), and hence the normal QRS complex (Diagram A of Fig. 205, and Fig. 206).

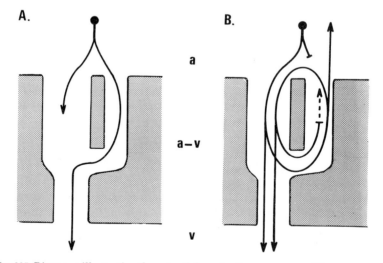

Fig. 205. Diagrams illustrating the potential conduction sequences of the Lown-Ganong-Levine syndrome. (A) illustrates the basic rapid conduction sequence; (B) illustrates the potential reciprocating conduction sequence.

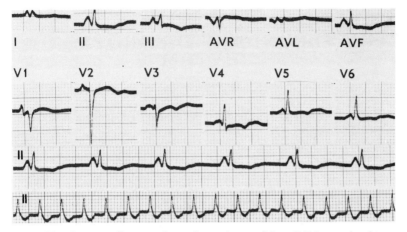

Fig. 206. The electrocardiograms shows the syndrome of short P–R interval and normal QRS complex—the L.G.L. syndrome. Note: 1. Normal sinus rhythm. This is shown in the top rhythm strip (standard lead II). The P–P intervals measure 0.84 sec, reflecting a rate of 71 beats per minute. 2. Tall P waves. The P waves in Standard lead II are 3 mm in height and tend to be peaked. This may reflect right atrial enlargement. 3. Short P–R interval. The P–R interval measures 0.10 sec. There is no P–R segment, i.e. the P wave occupies the whole of the P–R interval. 4. The QRS complexes are normal. 5. Supraventricular reciprocating tachycardia. This is shown in the lower rhythm strip (standard lead II). The R–R intervals measure 0.28 sec, reflecting a rate of 214 beats per minute. The QRS complexes are the same as those seen during normal sinus rhythm (upper rhythm strip), thereby reflecting the supraventricular origin of the tachycardia. There is 1:1 conduction and the P′ waves deform the S-T segment.

As in the W-P-W. syndrome, the presence of a by-pass facilitates reciprocal return to the atria. The returning impulse may initiate a reciprocating tachycardia (Diagrams B and F of Fig. 194 and B of Fig. 205).

REFERENCES

1 ROSENBAUM F. F., HECHT H. H., WILSON F. N. & JOHNSTON F. D. (1945) The potential variations of the thorax and the oesophagus in anomalous atrioventricular excitation (Wolff-Parkinson-White syndrome). *Amer. Heart J.* **29**, 281.
2 SCHAMROTH L. (1975) Observations on the QRS complex in the Wolff-Parkinson-White syndrome. Recent Advances in Ventricular Conduction. Ed. by M. Cerqueira-Gomes. *Adv. Cardiol.* **14**, 210. Karger, Basel.
3 SODI-PALLARES D. & CALDER R. M. (1956) *New Bases of Electrocardiography*. St. Louis: C. V. Mosby Co.
4 WOLFF L., PARKINSON L. & WHITE P. D. (1930) Bundle branch block with short P–R interval in healthy young people prone to paroxysmal tachycardia. *Amer. Heart J.* **5**, 685.

SECTION 4

THE SECONDARY DISORDERS OF RHYTHM

Escape Rhythms
A-V Dissociation
Ventricular Fusion Complexes
Phasic Aberrant Ventricular Conduction

Chapter 22
Escape Rhythms

The heart has many potential pacemakers which are situated in the sino-atrial node, the atria, the A-V node, and the ventricles. Each pacemaker has its own inherent rate and cycle length. The more distal the pacemaker is situated from the S-A node, the slower its automaticity or inherent discharge rate. However, it is only the

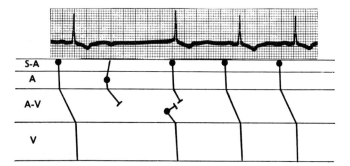

Fig. 207. Electrocardiogram (Standard lead I) showing A-V nodal escape following a blocked atrial extrasystole. Note (a) the blocked atrial extrasystole is reflected by the bizarre, inverted and premature P′ wave which occurs after the first conducted beat, and which is not followed by a QRS complex; (b) the A-V nodal escape beat is reflected by the QRS complex following the blocked atrial extrasystole which is normal in shape and is not preceded by a P wave; (c) the sinus impulse following the extrasystole occurs synchronously with the A-V nodal escape beat. The sinus P wave is, therefore, hidden within the A-V nodal QRS complex.

244

fastest pacemaker—the pacemaker with the highest automaticity (usually the S-A node)—that is normally in control in the heart, since its impulses reach the slower subsidiary pacemakers before they have an opportunity to 'fire' and discharge or abolish their immature impulses prematurely. The cycle of the subsidiary pacemaker must then begin anew, i.e. from the moment of its passive discharge by the faster pacemaker. This reset ectopic cycle will, however, again be anticipated and hence interrupted by the next sinus impulse. This ensures that there is only one pacemaker in control of the heart. At times, however, the impulses from the fastest pacemaker fail to reach the slower subsidiary pacemaker. This may be due to block in the conduction of the sinus impulses or a slowing of the sinus rate. When this occurs, the impulses from a slower potential subsidiary pacemaker (in the atria, A-V node or ventricles) have an opportunity to reach maturity and are thus able to discharge spontaneously. This spontaneous discharge of a slower subsidiary pacemaker is known as an *escape beat* (Figs. 207 and 211), since the slower pacemaker has so to speak 'escaped' from the influence of the faster pacemaker. If the

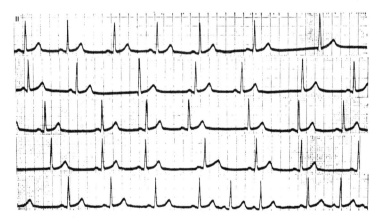

Fig. 208. The electrocardiogram (a continuous strip of Standard lead II) shows: 1. *Sinus rhythm with sinus arrhythmia. Periods of sinus bradycardia during the bradycardic phase of the sinus arrhythmia.* 2. *A-V nodal escape.* The long pauses resulting from the sinus bradycardia are terminated by A-V nodal escape beats. These escape beats are represented by the last QRS complex in the top strip, the third and sixth QRS complexes in the second strip, the second and fifth QRS complexes in the third strip, and the first QRS complex in the fourth strip. These escape beats have QRS complexes of identical contour to those of the conducted sinus beats. The near synchronous P waves of the sinus rhythm are dissociated from the QRS complexes and are superimposed upon the QRS complexes of the escape beats, or occur just before the escape beats with a shorter P to R interval.

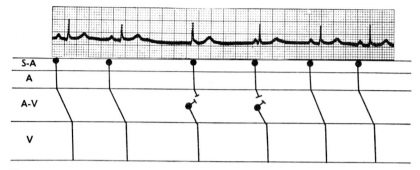

Fig. 209. Electrocardiogram (Standard lead II) showing two A-V nodal escape beats following sinus bradycardia during the bradycardic phase of sinus arrhythmia. Black dots indicate impulse origin. S-A = sino-atrial level; A = atrial level; A-V = A-V nodal level; V = ventricular level.

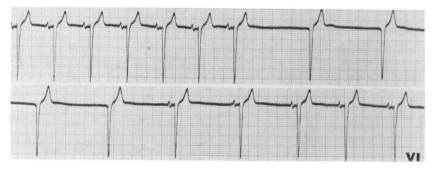
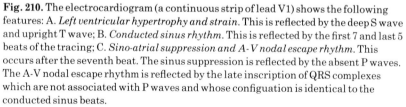

Fig. 210. The electrocardiogram (a continuous strip of lead V1) shows the following features: A. *Left ventricular hypertrophy and strain*. This is reflected by the deep S wave and upright T wave; B. *Conducted sinus rhythm*. This is reflected by the first 7 and last 5 beats of the tracing; C. *Sino-atrial suppression and A-V nodal escape rhythm*. This occurs after the seventh beat. The sinus suppression is reflected by the absent P waves. The A-V nodal escape rhythm is reflected by the late inscription of QRS complexes which are not associated with P waves and whose configuation is identical to the conducted sinus beats.

subsidiary pacemaker is able to discharge for two or more beats, the rhythm is known as *escape rhythm* (Figs. 208, 209, 210 and 212).

Basic causes

Failure of sinus impulses to reach the slower subsidiary pacemaker may be due to two basic disturbances:

A. *Primary depression of the sinus pacemaker*. This is a depression

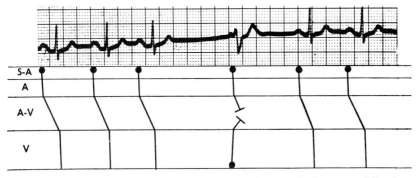

Fig. 211. Electrocardiogram (Standard lead II) showing ventricular escape following the bradycardic phase of the sinus arrhythmia. Note (*a*) sinus rhythm with marked sinus arrhythmia; (*b*) first-degree A-V block: the P–R interval measures 0.23 sec; (*c*) the bizarre QRS complex occurs late and follows a pause; (*d*) the ectopic beat near-synchronously with the sinus P wave resulting in momentary A-V dissociation.

or slowing of impulse formation within the S-A node as reflected by sinus bradycardia (Figs. 210, 211, 212 and 213).

B. *Conduction failure of the sinus impulses.* Failure of the faster sinus impulses to reach the slower subsidiary pacemaker may also be due to a conduction disturbance which prevents the sinus impulse from reaching the slower subsidiary pacemaker, e.g. S-A block and second- or third-degree A-V block (Figs. 182 to 187).

Thus, escape rhythm is a *consequence of* primary failure of the sinus rhythm and, as such, is never a primary diagnosis.

Note. A demand electrical pacemaker is, in effect, an artifical escape beat or rhythm. This is because the pacemaker is so designed that it will only stimulate if it does not sense any electrical activity—the QRS complex—for a set period.

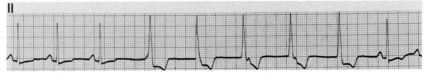

Fig. 212. Electrocardiogram (Standard lead II) showing a basic sinus rhythm with sinus arrhythmia, as reflected by the first 3 and the last 2 beats. A bradycardic phase of the sinus arrhythmia occurs after the third conducted beat. This is followed by a ventricular escape rhythm as reflected by the bizarre QRS complexes. The R–R intervals of this escape rhythm measure 0.92 sec, representing a rate of 65 per minute. The escape rhythm is dissociated from the near-synchronous sinus P waves which are superimposed upon and deform the QRS complex or the S-T segment.

Electrocardiographic manifestations

1. The escape beat occurs *late*, i.e. it follows an interval that is longer than the dominant cycle length.

2. Atrial escape is characterized by the late inscription of an abnormal P wave—a P' deflection (Fig. 213).

3. A-V nodal escape is characterized by the late inscription of an A-V nodal beat (Figs. 207, 208, 209 and 210).

4. Ventricular escape is characterized by the late inscription of a bizarre QRS complex of an ectopic ventricular beat (Figs. 211 and 212).

SIGNIFICANCE

Escape beats only occur as a result of primary pacemaker default. They are, therefore, a secondary phenomenon, and do not have any primary significance. Thus, the significance of escape rhythm is the significance of the sinus bradycardia, S-A block or A-V block which leads to the escape. Escape rhythm is never a primary diagnosis.

Chapter 23
A-V Dissociation

A-V dissociation is a *non-specific* or *generic* term which may be applied to any rhythm where the atria and the ventricles are activated independently, i.e. by two pacemakers; the atria being completely or dominantly governed by one pacemaker, and the ventricles completely or dominantly by another. A-V dissociation is not a primary disturbance, and the term, as such, is never a primary diagnosis (Pick, 1953[2]), for the condition always comes about as a result of another arrhythmic disturbance.

BASIC MECHANISMS

There are two basic mechanisms which may lead to A-V dissociation. These are:
  1. A disturbance of impulse formation.
  2. A disturbance of impulse conduction.

1. DISTURBANCES OF IMPULSE FORMATION

Disturbances of impulse formation may lead to A-V dissociation if they result in fortuitous, synchronous or near-synchronous discharge of supraventricular and ventricular pacemakers. When this occurs, the impulses from these pacemakers meet or 'collide'— usually within the A-V node, and impede each other's mutual progress. This mutual impedence is termed **interference,** for in an electrical sense, the impulses interfere with each other's conduction. The resulting dissociation is termed **'interference-dissociation'**.

EXAMPLES:

   A. *Ventricular or A-V nodal extrasystoles*, where the ventricular or A-V nodal discharge occurs at the same time as the sinus discharge (Figs. 157, 158 and 159).
   B. *Ventricular or A-V nodal tachycardia* which are complicated by interference. See section below on interference-dissociation.

C. *A-V nodal or ventricular escape beats* where the escaping focus discharges at the same time as the delayed sinus discharge (Figs. 207, 208, 209, 210, 211 and 212).

2. DISTURBANCES OF IMPULSE CONDUCTION

Complete A-V block or high-grade A-V block will lead to A-V dissociation since the sinus and subsidiary escape impulses (A-V nodal or ventricular) are prevented from 'invading' each other's territory.

INTERFERENCE-DISSOCIATION

There are two basic disturbances of *impulse formation* which may lead to interference-dissociation. These are:
     1. Late or delayed impulse formation.
     2. Early or accelerated impulse formation.

1. Late or delayed impulse formation leading to interference-dissociation

Interference-dissociation may be brought about by late or delayed impulse formation. For example, the advent of sinus bradycardia may result in a prolongation of the sinus cycle so that it approximates the cycle of a subsidiary A-V nodal or ventricular escape rhythm. When this occurs, the delayed sinus impulse will discharge synchronously with the escaping impulse. The two impulses then meet and interfere with each other's mutual progress, resulting in interference-dissociation (Figs. 207 to 212, and 214).

2. Premature or enhanced impulse formation leading to interference-dissociation

Interference-dissociation may be brought about by premature or enhanced impulse formation of a subsidiary A-V nodal or ventricular pacemaker, e.g. A-V nodal and ventricular extrasystoles (Figs. 153, 154, 157, 158 and 159), idionodal tachycardia (Fig. 156), extrasystolic A-V nodal tachycardia (Fig. 155), idioventricular tachycardia (Figs. 169 and 170), extrasystolic ventricular tachycardia (Figs. 165 and 167). When this occurs, the subsidiary A-V nodal or ventricular cycles may be so shortened that they approximate the sinus cycle. Consequently, both the sinus and subsidiary pacemakers discharge

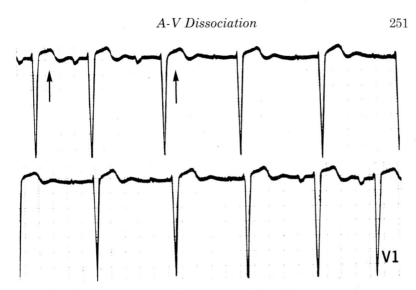

Fig. 213. The electrocardiogram (a continuous strip of lead V1) shows the following features: 1. *Basic sinus rhythm with sinus arrhythmia.* This is evident from the first 3 and last 2 beats. 2. *Atrial escape.* This follows carotid sinus compression (applied between the arrows), and is reflected by the manifestation of different P waves which are bizarre and of low amplitude. The P′–P′ interval measures 1.12 sec, representing a rate of 54 per minute. 3. *Left atrial enlargement.* This is evident from the marked terminal negativity of the sinus P waves. 4. *Left ventricular hypertrophy and strain.* This is evident from the deep S waves and the elevated S-T segments and T waves.

synchronously or near-synchronously, and their impulses will meet and interfere with each other's mutual progress within the A-V node.

Note. A-V dissociation will also be facilitated with enhanced subsidiary rhythms if, in addition, there is retrograde A-V block. When this occurs, the faster subsidiary rhythm can co-exist with a much slower sinus rhythm.

CAPTURE BEATS

When interference-dissociation occurs between sinus rhythm and a faster subsidiary (ventricular or A-V nodal) rhythm, the mutual impedance or interference occurs within the A-V node. The ventricular or A-V nodal impulses cannot be conducted retrogradely to the atria as a result of upper A-V nodal refractoriness consequent to partial penetration of the sinus impulses into the A-V node; and the sinus impulses cannot be conducted anterogradely to the ventricles as a result of lower A-V nodal refractoriness consequent to partial retrograde penetration of the ventricular impulses into the A-V node.

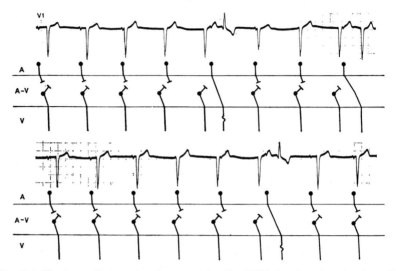

Fig. 214. Electrocardiogram (continuous strip of lead V1) showing *sinus bradycardia*
with *A-V dissociation* from an *idionodal escape rhythm.* The P waves of the slower
sinus rhythm are dissociated from the QRS complexes of the *relatively* faster
idionodal rhythm. The impulses from these two rhythms meet within the A-V node
and interfere with, or impede, each other's mutual progress, thereby resulting in A-V
dissociation. Since the sinus rhythm is slower than the idionodal rhythm the P
waves 'encroach' progressively on the QRS complexes, and then 'overtake'—are
recorded after—the QRS complexes. When the sinus impulse occurs after the
idionodal beat it may reach the A-V node when it is no longer refractory consequent
to activation by the idionodal impulse. When this occurs, the sinus impulse is
conducted to, and momentarily activates or captures, the ventricles. There are three
capture beats in the recording (diagrammed). The first and third capture beats are
conducted with phasic aberrant ventricular conduction resulting in bizarre QRS
complexes which are related to the preceding P waves. The second capture beat is
conducted with a longer P–R interval thereby resulting in normal intraventricular
conduction, since both bundle branches have adequate time for recovery. The QRS
complex of the normally conducted capture beat resembles the QRS complexes of the
idionodal rhythm thus establishing the A-V nodal origin of the idionodal rhythm.

However, as the two pacemakers discharge asynchronously, the
slower sinus discharge occurs progressively later in relation to the
A-V nodal or ventricular discharge, i.e. the sinus P wave 'falls'
further and further away from the QRS complex of the subsidiary
rhythm. The sinus impulse may thus eventually reach the A-V node
when it is no longer refractory. It is then able to penetrate the A-V
node and be conducted to and activate the ventricles. This momentary activation of the ventricles by the sinus impulse during A-V
dissociation is known as a **ventricular capture beat**—for the sinus

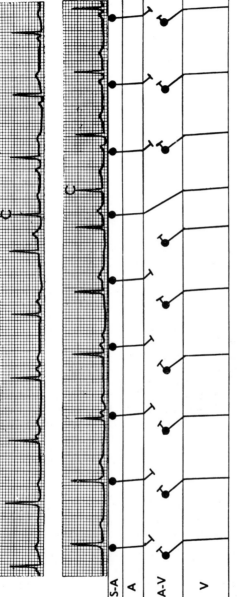

Fig. 215. Electrocardiogram (continuous recording of Standard lead II; the diagram refers to the bottom strip only) showing interference-dissociation. The sinus discharge is slower than the A-V nodal discharge, i.e. the P–P intervals are longer than the R–R intervals; the P waves are thus unrelated to, or dissociated from, the QRS complexes. The first P wave in the lower strip is hidden within the QRS complex; the second P wave deforms the terminal part of the QRS complex; subsequent P waves occur progressively further away from the QRS complexes. The first sinus discharge (lower strip) find the A-V node refractory; the sixth sinus discharge occurs at a relatively longer interval from the preceding QRS complex and thus finds the A-V node recovered; it is, therefore, conducted to the ventricles resulting in a premature QRS complex—the capture beat (labelled C).

impulse momentarily captures the ventricles which are under control of the subsidiary pacemaker. The capture beat occurs before the next scheduled subsidiary beat and is, therefore, an *early* beat. And this early beat must be related to a preceding sinus P wave (Figs. 167, 214, 215 and 229).

Electrocardiographically the rhythm manifests with P waves which bear no relationship to the QRS complexes. And as the sinus rhythm is slower than the subsidiary ventricular rhythm, the P–P intervals will be longer than the R–R intervals. As a result, the P waves will 'overtake' the QRS complexes, i.e. the 'P–R' interval becomes progressively shorter. The P wave then becomes super-imposed upon the QRS complex and eventually occurs after the QRS complex. And when the P wave falls sufficiently far beyond the QRS complex, the sinus impulse is conducted to the ventricles resulting in an earlier QRS complex—the ventricular capture beat.

Note: A-V dissociation should always be suspected when the P–R intervals become progressively shorter.

For further details, the reader is referred to the reviews of Marriott (1958)[1] and Schott (1959).[3]

REFERENCES

1 MARRIOTT H. J. J. (1958) A-V dissociation: a re-appraisal. *Amer. J. Cardiol.* **2,** 586.
2 PICK A. (1963) A-V dissociation. A proposal for a comprehensive classification and consistent terminology. *Amer. Heart J.* **66,** 147.
3 SCHOTT A. (1959) Atrioventricular dissociation with and without interference. *Progr. Cardiovasc. Dis.* **2,** 444.

Chapter 24
Ventricular Fusion Complexes

A ventricular fusion complex is recorded when two impulses invade the ventricles simultaneously (Fig. 216). Each impulse activates part of the ventricles and the resulting QRS complex has a configuration that is between that of the 'pure' QRS complex of the ectopic beat: the complex resulting from activation by the ectopic impulse only, and the 'pure' QRS complex of the sinus beat: the QRS complex resulting from activation by the sinus impulse only. This 'inbetween' QRS complex is known as a *fusion complex* (syns: summation complex, combination beat). It is clear, therefore, that ventricular fusion can only be diagnosed if all three forms of QRS complexes are present in the same lead of the same tracing. Thus, the lead must reflect:

1. The 'pure' ectopic QRS complex
2. The 'pure' sinus QRS complex
3. The intermediate fusion complex.

It should, if possible, also be shown that the timing of the two impulses is such that they do, in fact, discharge synchronously at the time the fusion complex is recorded. For example, the timing of a parasystolic beat giving rise to the fusion complex must be calculated to coincide with that of a conducted sinus beat (Chapter 16, Fig. 174).

THE VARIABILITY IN THE FORM OF THE VENTRICULAR FUSION COMPLEX

The modification of the QRS complex by fusion will depend upon the relative contribution of the supraventricular and ventricular impulses to ventricular activation. If the contribution is dominantly by the supraventricular impulse (Diagram E of Fig. 216), the fusion complex will resemble the 'pure' sinus QRS complex. If the contribution is dominantly by the ectopic impulse, the fusion will resemble the 'pure' ectopic QRS complex (Diagram D of Fig. 216). If the contributions by both impulses to ventricular activation are approximately the same (Diagram C of Fig. 216), the QRS complex will have a configuration that is more or less between that of the 'pure' ectopic and the 'pure' sinus QRS complexes. Thus, in any one tracing there is

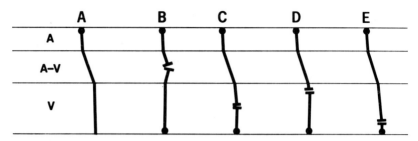

Fig. 216. Diagram illustrating: (A) a normally conducted sinus beat; (B) an ectopic ventricular beat with dissociation and interference from the near-synchronous sinus impulse within the A-V junction; (C), (D) and (E) ectopic ventricular beats with dissociation and interference from the near-synchronous sinus impulse within the ventricles, resulting in various degrees of ventricular fusion.

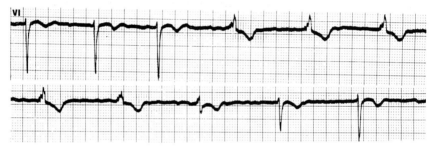

Fig. 217. The electrocardiogram (a continuous strip of lead V1) shows: 1. *Atrial fibrillation*. This is evident from (*a*) the irregular baseline due to the distortion of the 'f' waves, and (*b*) the irregular ventricular response. 2. *A slow ventricular response*. The presence of high-grade A-V block—a slow ventricular response—is evidenced by the first two relatively long cycles of 1.11 sec. and 0.98 sec respectively, reflecting a ventricular rate of approximately 60 beats per minute. 3. *Ventricular escape rhythm*. This is represented by the fourth and ensuing QRS complexes. The R–R intervals of this escape rhythm measure 1.16 sec, 1.18 sec, 1.17 sec, 1.21 sec, 1.24 sec and 1.23 sec respectively, representing a rate of about 50 beats per minute. 4. *Ventricular fusion complexes*. These are reflected by the last four QRS complexes whose configuration is in between that of the 'pure' conducted supraventricular complex and the 'pure' escape complex. The configuration of these complexes varies depending upon the relative contribution of each pacemaking impulse to activation of the ventricles. The first two fusion complexes have the greatest resemblance to the 'pure' ectopic ventricular rhythm, and this reflects a dominant contribution by the ectopic ventricular pacemaker (as represented by Diagram D of Fig. 216). The last two QRS fusion complexes bear the closest resemblance to the conducted supraventricular complexes, and thus reflect a dominant contribution from the supraventricular impulses (as represented by Diagram E of Fig. 216). Note that even the last QRS complex is probably a fusion complex, since although it is virtually the same as the conducted supraventricular complex, the S wave is not as deep, and the T wave is not quite the same.

a tendency to variability in the QRS configuration of the fusion complexes (Fig. 217).

The diagnosis of ventricular fusion will, therefore, be substantiated by marked variation in the form of the ventricular fusion QRS complexes (Fig. 217).

THE MECHANISMS OF VENTRICULAR FUSION

There are two possible mechanisms or forms of ventricular fusion complexes:

A. *Fusion due to interference-dissociation at the ventricular level*

Interference-dissociation at the ventricular level is due to simultaneous invasion of the ventricles by supraventricular and ectopic ventricular impulses. This is the common form of ventricular fusion complex, and is the form considered above.

Abnormal rhythms giving rise to this form of fusion complex are:
1.   Ventricular parasystole (page 202).
2.   End-diastolic ventricular extrasystoles (page 182).
3.   Incomplete capture beats during ventricular tachycardia (page 191).

B. *Fusion due to the Wolff-Parkinson-White syndrome*

The fusion complex of the Wolff-Parkinson-White syndrome is due to simultaneous invasion of the ventricles by a single supraventricular impulse, whose activation front divides into two. Each of these subsidiary activation fronts is conducted to the ventricles through a different A-V pathway, consequently activating different parts of the ventricular chamber. This manifestation is discussed in greater detail in the chapter on 'The Wolff-Parkinson-White Syndrome' (Chapter 21).

Chapter 25
Phasic Aberrant Ventricular Conduction

Thus the spread of the excitation wave to the ventricles, considered together, is abnormal by reason of a defect in a chief distributing channel; consequently I term the resultant contractions 'aberrant', for they are the product of impulses which have gone astray.

THOMAS LEWIS

An isolated, bizarre QRS complex, or a periodic succession of bizarre QRS complexes, is not necessarily the result of ectopic ventricular discharge but may be due to *temporary* abnormal intraventricular conduction (bundle branch block) of a supraventricular impulse. This isolated form of bundle branch block occurs during rhythm that otherwise shows normal intraventricular conduction. Lewis (1912)[2] termed this condition **aberrant ventricular conduction** and defined it as the abnormal intraventricular conduction of a supraventricular impulse. Strict interpretation of this definition, however, makes it applicable to both the temporary *and* permanent forms of abnormal intraventricular conduction. To define these conditions more accurately, the term **phasic** aberrant ventricular conduction was introduced to distinguish the temporary form from the **nonphasic** or permanent form of aberrant ventricular conduction (Schamroth & Chesler, 1963[9]).

Aberrant ventricular conduction results in a bizarre QRS complex resembling left or right bundle branch block. In phasic aberrant ventricular conduction these bizarre QRS complexes occur during rhythms which otherwise show normal intraventricular conduction. Thus, phasic aberrant ventricular conduction may mimic the bizarre complexes found in ventricular ectopic rhythms, e.g. paroxysmal—extrasystolic—ventricular tachycardia. The recognition of phasic aberrant ventricular conduction is thus of major clinical import, since the differentiation of supraventricular from ventricular rhythms affects both prognosis and treatment.

MECHANISM

Phasic aberrant ventricular conduction may complicate any supraventricular rhythm, viz. sinus rhythm, A-V nodal rhythm, atrial and A-V nodal extrasystoles, paroxysmal atrial and A-V nodal tachycardias, atrial flutter and atrial fibrillation. The disturbance is dependent upon:

1. **Unequal refractory periods of the bundle branches.**
2. **Critical premature impulse formation.**
3. **The length of the preceding R–R interval.**

When the refractory periods of the bundle branches are equal (Fig. 172A), an impulse which occurs relatively late (at position 2) will find both bundle branches fully recovered and will be conducted with normal intraventricular conduction. An impulse which occurs very early (at position 1) will find both bundles refractory and will be blocked, and there will be no intraventricular conduction.

When the refractory periods of the bundle branches are unequal (Fig. 218B), an impulse which occurs relatively late (at position 3) will be conducted with normal intraventricular conduction. An impulse which occurs very early—at position 1—will be blocked; an impulse which occurs with a critical prematurity—at position 2, i.e. between positions 1 and 3, will find one bundle branch recovered and the other refractory—it will thus be conducted down one bundle branch only, resulting in the bizarre QRS pattern of bundle branch block. It is usually the left bundle branch that recovers first and thus phasic aberrant ventricular conduction commonly, though not invariably, results in a right bundle branch block pattern. Hence it will be seen that **unequal refractory periods are essential to the**

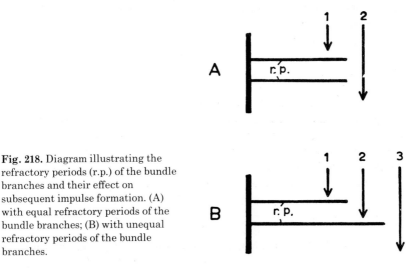

Fig. 218. Diagram illustrating the refractory periods (r.p.) of the bundle branches and their effect on subsequent impulse formation. (A) with equal refractory periods of the bundle branches; (B) with unequal refractory periods of the bundle branches.

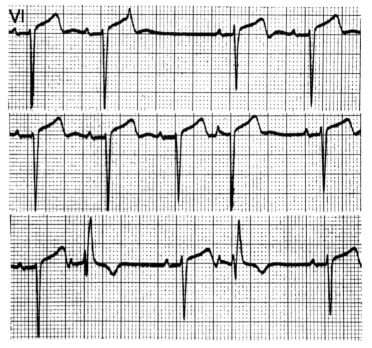

Fig. 219. Electrocardiogram (non-continuous strips of lead V1) illustrating:

A. *Top strip.* A blocked—non-conducted—atrial extrasystole. The premature bizarre P wave is superimposed upon the T wave of the second sinus beat.

B. *Middle strip.* A normally conducted atrial extrasystole. The fourth P wave is premature and bizarre. It is, however, *relatively* late (compare with top strip) and is, therefore, conducted normally.

C. *Bottom strip.* Atrial extrasystoles conducted with phasic aberrant, ventricular conduction. The second and fourth P waves are premature, bizarre, and followed by QRS complexes showing the right bundle branch block pattern of phasic aberrant ventricular conduction. Note the timing of these extrasystoles is in between the extrasystoles of the top and middle strips.

occurrence of phasic aberrant ventricular conduction, and that the phenomenon is **favoured by critically timed premature impulses**—the earlier the impulse, within limits, the more likely it is to find one of the bundle branches refractory.

These phenomena are illustrated in Figs. 219, 220, 221, 224, 225, 226, 227 and 237. Fig. 219 shows atrial extrasystoles: very early extrasystoles are blocked; late extrasystoles are conducted with normal intraventricular conduction, extrasystoles intermediate in timing are conducted with aberration. Fig. 220 is an example of

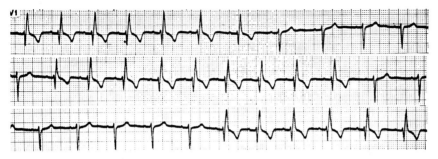

Fig. 220. Electrocardiogram (continuous strip of lead V1) showing sinus rhythm with bundle branch block dependent upon critical rate. There is slight sinus arrhythmia. The shorter cycles are associated with right bundle branch block conduction—a manifestation of phasic aberrant ventricular conduction. The longer cycles are associated with normal intraventricular conduction.

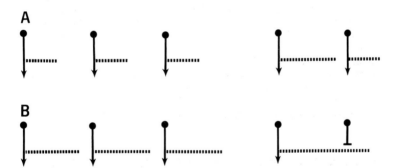

Fig. 221. Electrocardiogram showing atrial extrasystoles (marked with arrows) conducted with different degrees of aberration.

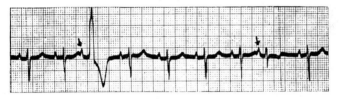

Fig. 222. Diagrams illustrating the Ashman phenomenon. The dotted lines represent the refractory periods following each conducted beat. When the rhythm is regular, as reflected by the first 3 beats in each diagram, the refractory periods remain regular. When the cycle suddenly increases (as illustrated by the cycle between the third and fourth beats in both A and B), the ensuing refractory period lengthens. When the basic refractory period is already long or relatively long (as illustrated in B), the additional lengthening resulting from the Ashman phenomenon may result in the block on an ensuing impulse.

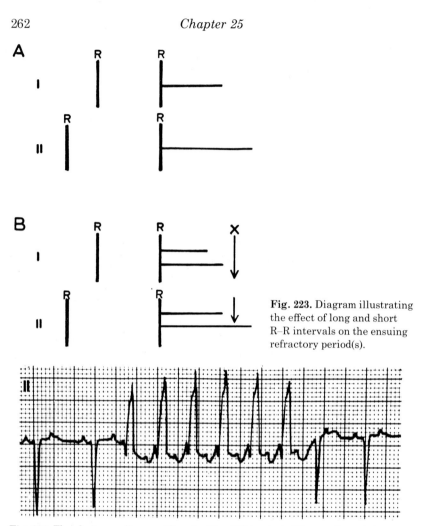

Fig. 223. Diagram illustrating the effect of long and short R–R intervals on the ensuing refractory period(s).

Fig. 224. The electrocardiogram (Standard lead II) begins with a conducted sinus impulse. This is followed by a blocked atrial extrasystole. The P′ wave of the atrial extrasystole is superimposed upon the T wave of the sinus beat. The coupling interval of the atrial extrasystole (P–P′ interval) measures 0.25 sec. The extrasystolic impulse is very premature and, therefore, encounters refractory A-V nodal tissue. The extrasystole is followed by another conducted sinus beat which in turn is followed by a further atrial extrasystole. This atrial extrasystole, however, occurs slightly later: the coupling interval (P–P′ interval) measures 0.29 sec. This impulse finds the A-V node and the left bundle branch responsive, and is consequently conducted to the ventricles with phasic aberrant ventricular conduction—a right bundle branch block pattern. This is followed by a paroxysm of successive atrial extrasystoles—an extrasystolic atrial tachycardia—which is conducted with the same form of aberration. *Note*: Every bizarre QRS complex is related to a preceding P′ wave.

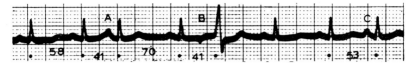

Fig. 225. Electrocardiogram showing three atrial extrasystoles (labelled A, B and C). Extrasystole C occurs relatively late and is thus normally conducted. Extrasystoles A and B result in QRS complexes which occur at the same interval (0.41 sec) from the preceding sinus beat; A is normally conducted as it is preceded by a relatively short R–R interval (0.58 sec); B is conducted with aberration as it is preceded by a relatively long R–R interval (0.70 sec). All time intervals are indicated in hundredths of a second.

intermittent bundle branch block dependent upon critical rate (Vesell, 1941[12]; Shearn & Rytand, 1953[10]). With a relatively slow heart rate, the sinus impulses find both bundle branches fully recovered and are normally conducted (mechanism illustrated by position 3 in Diagram B of Fig. 218). With an increase in heart rate, the sinus impulses find the left bundle branch refractory and the right bundle branch responsive; and are, therefore, conducted with the right bundle branch block pattern of phasic aberrant ventricular conduction (mechanism illustrated by position 2 in Diagram B of Fig. 172).

The effect of cycle length on refractoriness: the Ashman Phenomenon

The significance of the preceding R–R interval

The duration of the refractory period is directly proportional to the

STD. 2

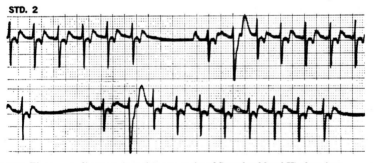

Fig. 226. Electrocardiogram (continuous strip of Standard lead II) showing paroxysms of supraventricular tachycardia (a form of reciprocal rhythm with retrograde atrial activation). Note that only the second QRS complex of each paroxysm is conducted with aberration; this is because it is only the second atrial impulse of each paroxysm that is preceded by a long R–R interval.

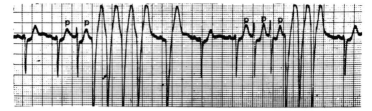

Fig. 227. Electrocardiogram showing paroxysms of atrial tachycardia conducted with aberration. The P waves (labelled) are seen before the bizarre QRS complexes at the beginning of each paroxysm; they are superimposed on the preceding T waves. Note the increasing abnormality of the QRS complexes as the rate speeds up. P waves cannot be distinguished during the 'full-blown' established tachycardia and the paroxysm then resembles ventricular tachycardia.

length of the preceding R–R interval (Figs. 222 and 223). With a long preceding R–R interval the subsequent refractory period will be relatively long (illustrated in Fig. 222 and Diagram A II of Fig. 223); with a shorter preceding R–R interval the subsequent refractory period will be relatively shorter (illustrated in Fig. 222 and Diagram A I of Fig. 223). In other words, the refractory period shortens with tachycardia and lengthens with bradycardia (Trendelenburg, 1903[11]; Mines, 1913[7]; Lewis, Drury & Bulger, 1921[3]). Thus, when there is a sudden lengthening of the cycle length, as may occur, for example, during atrial fibrillation, marked sinus arrhythmia and a blocked atrial extrasystole, there is a sudden prolongation of the ensuing refractory period. And this may result in a delay, or block in the conduction of the ensuing impulse. This is known as the Ashman Phenomenon.[1] The same principle applies in the presence of unequal refractory periods of the bundle branches. When the preceding R–R interval is relatively short, the subsequent refractory periods of the bundle branches will be relatively short (illustrated in Diagram B I of Fig. 223). When this occurs, an early beat—X—will find both bundle branches recovered and will be conducted normally. With a relatively long preceding R–R interval the subsequent refractory periods of the bundle branches will be relatively long (illustrated in Diagram B II of Fig. 223) and an early impulse—X—(of the same prematurity as illustrated in Diagram B I)—will now find one bundle branch refractory and is, therefore, conducted with ventricular aberration. **Phasic aberrant ventricular conduction is thus favoured by a long preceding R–R interval.** This is illustrated in Fig. 225. The tracing shows three atrial extrasystoles—A, B and C. Extrasystoles A and B result in identical R–R intervals (0.41 sec), yet extrasystole A is conducted normally whereas extrasystole B is conducted with ventricular aberration. This is because B is preceded by a long R–R interval (0.70 sec), whereas extrasystole A is preceded by a short R–R interval (0.58 sec).

This principle is also illustrated in Fig. 226 where *only the second beat* of a run of paroxysmal supraventricular tachycardia shows aberrant ventricular conduction—a pattern that may almost be regarded as a hallmark of phasic aberrant ventricular conduction. This occurs because only the second beat of the paroxysm is preceded by a long R–R interval, whereas the subsequent beats of the tachycardia are preceded by short R–R intervals. If, however, the second and subsequent beats occur *very* early, then all the beats may be conducted with ventricular aberration (Fig. 227). The same principle may be evident in cases of atrial flutter with alternating 4:1 and 2:1 A-V block (see page 275 and Figs. 237 and 238).

THE DIFFERENTIATION OF ECTOPIC VENTRICULAR RHYTHMS FROM SUPRAVENTRICULAR RHYTHMS WITH PHASIC ABERRANT VENTRICULAR CONDUCTION

The differentiation of ectopic ventricular rhythms from supraventricular rhythms conducted with phasic aberrant ventricular conduction is based primarily on four basic principles:

1. The relationship of the abnormal QRS complex to a preceding atrial event.
2. The identification and appraisal of capture beats.
3. The recognition of characteristic QRS morphological appearances.
4. The presence or absence of an attempt at a compensatory pause.

1. *The relationship of the abnormal QRS complex to a preceding atrial event*

Phasic aberrant ventricular conduction reflects the abnormal intraventricular conduction of a supraventricular impulse, and is thus usually preceded by an atrial event, a P or P′ wave. For example, a bizarre QRS complex preceded by a premature and bizarre P′ wave usually represents an atrial extrasystole conducted with phasic aberrant ventricular conduction (Figs. 219, 220, 221 and 224); whereas a bizarre QRS complex that is not preceded by a related P wave usually represents ventricular ectopy. Thus, the recognition of a related preceding P or P′ wave favours a diagnosis of aberrant ventricular conduction.

Preceding and related atrial activity, however, may not always be evident electrocardiographically. There is, for example, no related preceding recognizable atrial activity in cases of atrial fibrillation. An A-V nodal or junctional extrasystole may also be conducted with aberration, and yet have no preceding atrial event. It may also be very difficult to identify the atrial deflections in a series of rapidly inscribed bizarre QRS complexes of a paroxysmal atrial tachycardia. Furthermore, even if the P waves and the QRS complexes in a tachyarrhythmia are identified, the relationship of the P′ waves to

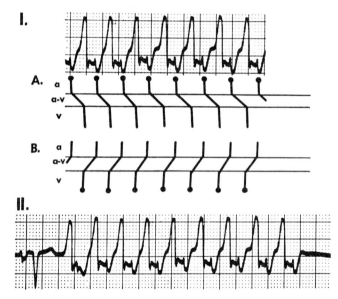

Fig. 228. Electrocardiograms (lead V1). Electrocardiogram I shows a tachycardia which is reflected by the bizarre QRS complexes. Each QRS complex is related to a bizarre P′ wave. However, it is impossible to tell whether this represents extrasystolic atrial tachycardia with phasic aberrant ventricular conduction (as illustrated in Diagram A) or extrasystolic ventricular tachycardia with retrograde A-V conduction (as illustrated in Diagram B). Definitive diagnosis is possible when the beginning of the tachycardia is observed (Electrocardiogram II). The first bizarre QRS complex is now seen to be followed by a P′ wave, i.e. it is not related to a preceding P′ wave. This, as well as the bizarre, monophasic form of the QRS complex, establishes the ventricular origin of the tachycardia (as illustrated in Diagram I B).

the bizarre QRS complexes may not be clear unless the beginning of the tachyarrhythmia is observed. For example, the P′ wave may, during a tachyarrhythmia, represent an ectopic atrial origin, or it may reflect retrograde atrial activation from a ventricular or A-V nodal impulse.

This is illustrated in Fig. 228. Electrocardiogram 1 reveals a close relationship between the P′ deflections and the bizarre QRS complexes: every QRS complex is related to a P′ deflection. This relationship, however, could represent (i) a ventricular tachycardia with retrograde conduction to the atria; every QRS complex would then be related to the ensuing P′ deflection (as illustrated in Diagram B of Fig. 228), or (ii) an ectopic atrial tachycardia with aberrant anterograde conduction to the ventricles; every QRS complex would then be related to the preceding P′ deflection (as illustrated in Diagram A of Fig. 228). The situation becomes clarified when the beginning of the paroxysm is observed (as shown in Diagram II of Fig. 228). It is now evident that the first abnormal QRS complex of the paroxysm is *followed* by the P′ deflection and the rhythm is, therefore, a ventricular tachycardia with retrograde conduction to the atria. The ventricular origin of the tachycardia is also suggested by the fact that the morphology of the QRS complexes is diphasic (almost monophasic) but not triphasic, and does not resemble either classic right or left bundle branch block (see below).

Note that A-V dissociation between P waves and bizarre QRS complexes does not necessarily connote ectopic ventricular origin since the bizarre QRS complexes may be the expression of an A-V nodal tachycardia with aberrant ventricular conduction. In such a circumstance the differentiation must be based on the morphology of the QRS complex (see below).

2. *The identification and appraisal of capture beats*

When a tachycardia with bizarre QRS complexes is complicated by capture beats, and the capture beat has a normal or near-normal narrow QRS configuration, the diagnosis of an ectopic ventricular tachycardia is strongly favoured (Fig. 229). This is because the supraventricular impulse must *ipso facto* follow a different course than that of the ectopic ventricular impulse. When the capture beat resembles the bizarre QRS pattern of the tachycardia, a diagnosis of supraventricular tachycardia with aberration is favoured (Fig. 155). This is because the course of activation of both the capturing and supraventricular ectopic impulse must be the same.

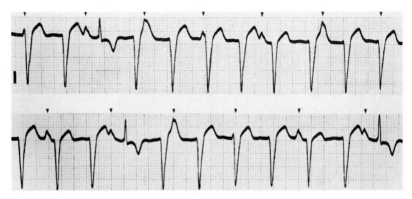

Fig. 229. The electrocardiogram (a continuous strip of Standard lead I) shows the following features: (*a*) Ventricular tachycardia. This is reflected by the bizarre dominantly negative QRS complexes. The R–R intervals measure 0.57 sec, representing a rate of 105 beats per minute. (*b*) Sinus bradycardia. This is reflected by the P waves (marked with small arrowheads), which are dissociated from the QRS complexes. The P–P intervals measure 1.02 sec representing a rate of 59 per minute. (*c*) Capture beats. These are reflected by the narrow upright QRS complexes and represent the momentary conduction to, and capture of, the ventricles. The capture beats are clearly related to a preceding P wave and are associated with a P–R interval of 0.26 sec. This takes place whenever a sinus impulse occurs at a critical interval from the preceding QRS complex. The impulse must fall outside the refractory period of the preceding beat; and conduction to the ventricles must occur before the next ectopic ventricular beat. The T wave of the capture beat is inverted, pointed, symmetrical and arrowhead in appearance, suggesting myocardia ischaemia.

The significance of partial ventricular capture: ventricular fusion

One of the best signs of ectopic ventricular origin is the presence of a ventricular fusion complex—a partial ventricular capture. This complex results from fortuitous concomitant activation of the ventricles by a supraventricular impulse and a ventricular impulse (Chapter 24).

3. *The recognition of characteristic QRS appearances*

Aberrant-ventricular conduction of supraventricular impulses tends to resemble right or left bundle branch block, which may further be modified by a complicating hemiblock. With ventricular ectopy, however, ventricular depolarization is usually completely bizarre. Because of this there are certain features in the QRS morphology which are strongly suggestive of either ventricular aberration or ventricular ectopy (Sandler & Marriott, 1965[8]; Marriott & Fogg, 1970[6]; Marriott 1972[5]). These are:

A. The significance of the initial QRS vector.

B. The significance of a triphasic, diphasic or monophasic configuration.

C. The significance of an rS or RS complex in lead V1.

D. The significance of the relative R and R′ amplitudes. The significance of the QRS 'Rabbit Ears'.

E. The significance of an initial q or Q wave in lead V1.

F. The significance of the concordant pattern.

G. The significance of a deepest QS complex in lead V4.

H. The significance of a QS complex in lead V6.

I. The significance of an rS or RS complex in lead V6.

J. The significance of a QS complex in Standard lead I.

K. The significance of the frontal plane QRS axis.

L. The variation in QRS configuration.

M. The duration of the QRS complex.

The first five of these features are best observed in lead V1 or lead MCL1 (Marriott and Fogg, 1970[6]; Fig. 230). This lead is formed by placing the positive pole of a bipolar monitoring lead on the lead V1 position, and the negative pole on the left shoulder just under the outer end of the clavicle (Fig. 230).

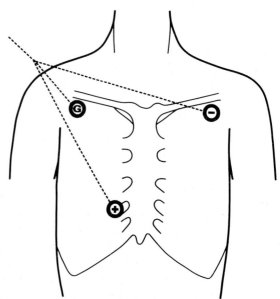

Fig. 230. Diagram illustrating the electrode placement of the MCL1 lead.[5]

In contrast to the usual monitoring bipolar lead placed on either side of the sternum, the MCL1 lead has the advantage that it does not interfere unduly with auscultation and other physical examination of the heart, it does not interfere with the administration of precordial electric shock, and it is less cumbersome for nursing the patient.

A. The significance of the initial vector. Most examples of phasic aberrant ventricular conduction reflect a right bundle branch block pattern. Right bundle branch block does not alter the initial vector of the QRS deflection (see Chapter 3 and Figs. 71 and 232). Hence the initial vectors of the QRS complex will tend to the same during both normal intraventricular conduction and phasic aberrant ventricular conduction (Figs. 219, 220 and 237). In ventricular ectopy, however, the initial vectors are usually markedly different (Fig. 228).

B. The significance of the triphasic configuration.[7] The QRS complex of right bundle branch block characteristically has a triphasic configuration, an rsR variant in lead V1 and a qRS variant in lead V6 (Diagram B of Fig. 71 and Fig. 232). The initial vectors (the

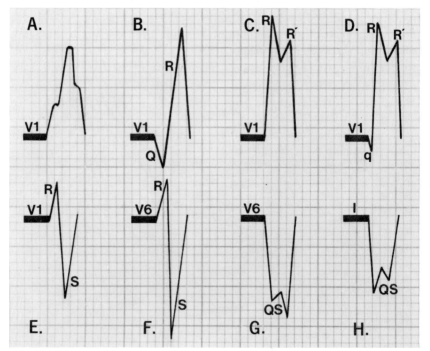

Fig. 231. Diagrams illustrating QRS forms in lead V1, V6 and Standard lead I, which favour ventricular ectopy.

rS deflection in right ventricular leads, and the qR deflection in left ventricular leads) are essentially unchanged. The right bundle branch merely results in the addition of a terminal deflection, an anterior and rightward directed vector. Hence, phasic aberrant ventricular conduction is usually associated with a triphasic configuration in lead V1. Similarly, a qRs complex in lead V6 is also an expression of right bundle branch block, and favours phasic aberrant ventricular conduction (Diagram B of Fig. 71 and Fig. 232). Ventricular ectopy, however, tends to have a monophasic or diphasic configuration in leads V1 or V6, a wide and bizarre dominantly upward or dominantly negative deflection with a notched apex or nadir (Fig. 232). Furthermore, the QRS complex of ventricular ectopy is completely bizarre, and does not resemble the classic forms of either right or left bundle branch block (Figs. 228, 231, 233, 234 and 235).

C. **The significance of an rS or RS complex in lead V1.** An rS or RS complex in lead V1 with a rather broad initial *r* or *R* wave usually indicates right ventricular ectopy (Fig. 231).

D. **The significance of the relative amplitude of the R and R′ deflections: the significance of the QRS 'Rabbit Ears'.** When lead V1 or lead MCL1 reflects a bizarre, dominantly upright QRS complex with a notched apex, and the initial deflection of the QRS complex, the *R* wave, is taller than the second deflection of the QRS

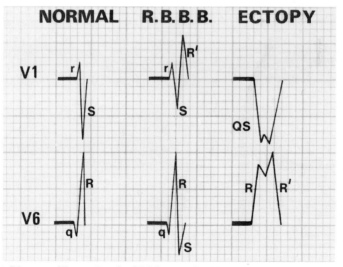

Fig. 232. Diagrams illustrating the QRS forms in leads V1 and V6 of normal intraventricular conduction, right bundle branch block and ventricular ectopy.

complex, the R' wave, ventricular ectopy is the most likely diagnosis (Figs. 231, 232 and 235). The notched upright QRS complex has been likened to a pair of rabbit ears,[3, 4] and when the first or left rabbit ear (viewing the rabbit from behind) of the QRS configuration is taller than the second rabbit ear, ventricular ectopy is the likely diagnosis. This may occasionally be preceded by a small initial q wave (Figs. 231, 232 and 235).

E. The significance of an initial q or Q wave in lead V1. An initial q wave or Q wave in lead V1 which is followed by an R wave is twice as common in cases of ectopic ventricular rhythm as in cases with phasic aberrant ventricular conduction.

F. The significance of the concordant pattern. If the electrocardiogram presents with a series of bizarre QRS complexes which are dominantly positive in *all* the precordial leads, ventricular ectopy is the most likely diagnosis (Fig. 233). The only other condition with a similar presentation is the Type A Wolff-Parkinson-White syndrome with atrial fibrillation, in which case the rhythm will be markedly irregular.

G. The significance of a deepest QS complex in lead V4. In left bundle branch block aberration, the QS complexes are always of greater depth in leads V1, V2 or V3 than in lead V4. The greatest

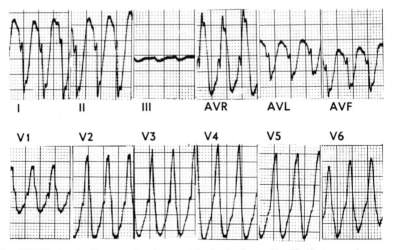

Fig. 233. Electrocardiogram showing ventricular tachycardia. The features of ventricular ectopy are evident from the following: (*a*) a positive precordial concordant pattern; (*b*) a bizarre QRS complex in lead V1 which resembles neither left nor right bundle branch block; (*c*) a QS complex in Standard lead I, and (*d*) a bizarre frontal plane QRS axis of − 150°.

magnitude is usually evident in lead V2. When, however, the QS depth is greatest in lead V4 the diagnosis is strongly suggestive of ventricular ectopy (Fig. 234).

H. The significance of a QS complex in lead V6. A QS complex—a wide, notched and entirely negative complex—in lead V6 usually connotes ventricular ectopy (Figs. 232 and 234).

I. The significance of an rS or RS complex in lead V6. An rS or RS complex in lead V6 is usually due to ventricular ectopy (Fig. 232). It may also be due to:

    (a) Right bundle branch block with left anterior hemiblock.

    (b) Marked right ventricular dominance.

    (c) Mirror-image dextrocardia.

Thus, when the features of the latter three conditions can be excluded (and this does not usually present any great difficulty), the presence of an rS or RS complex in lead V6 connotes ventricular ectopy.

J. The significance of a QS complex in Standard lead I. A QS configuration in Standard lead I (Figs. 229, 231, 233, 234 and 235) is very suggestive of ectopic ventricular origin provided anterior wall myocardial infarction can be excluded. Left bundle branch block aberration is always associated with positive deflections in Standard lead I. And while right bundle branch block aberration may be dominantly negative in Standard lead I, it is almost invariably preceded by a small initial r wave.

K. The significance of the mean frontal plane QRS axis. Phasic aberrant ventricular conduction is usually associated with a normal or near normal frontal plane QRS axis, for example, in the range of 0° to +90° or 100°, whereas ventricular ectopy is commonly

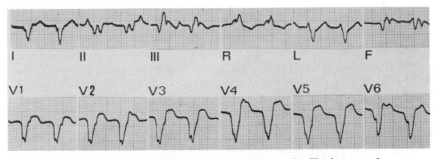

Fig. 234. Electrocardiogram showing ventricular tachycardia. The features of ventricular ectopy are evident from the following: (a) a negative precordial concordant pattern; (b) QS complex deeper in leads V4 and V5 than in lead V2; (c) QS complex in lead V6; (d) QS complex in Standard lead I; (e) bizarre frontal plane QRS axis of −150°. Note the presence of A-V dissociation, but seen in Standard lead II. This feature is not diagnostic of ventricular ectopy.

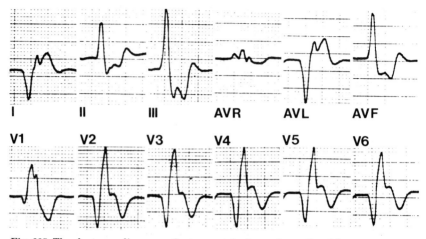

Fig. 235. The electrocardiogram reflects a ventricular tachycardia with retrograde A-V conduction to the atria. The 12-lead electrocardiogram reflects the following features of ventricular ectopy: (*a*) A positive precordial concordant pattern; (*b*) a qRR′ complex in lead V1 with the initial R deflection taller than the ensuing R′ deflection; (*c*) a QS complex in Standard lead I.

associated with a bizarre superiorly directed QRS axis in the region of 0° counterclockwise to − 180°. A frontal plane QRS axis in the "Northwest" region of − 90° counterclockwise to − 180° is especially suggestive, e.g. an axis of − 150° (Figs. 233 and 234).

L. **The variation in QRS configuration.** The QRS complexes in phasic aberrant ventricular conduction tend to be *multiform in character* with frequent fine gradations from normal to abnormal (Figs. 221, 225, 227 and 237). This is due to the fact that there are usually different degrees of prematurity—e.g. atrial fibrillation or atrial extrasystoles with different coupling intervals—which may result in varying degrees of aberration. This is in contrast to the situation with ectopic ventricular rhythm as manifest, for example, by ventricular extrasystoles which usually tend to have a uniform QRS configuration. Even if ventricular extrasystoles are multifocal, the electrocardiogram usually manifests with two or three fixed patterns. The fine gradations, as seen in phasic aberrant ventricular conduction, do not often occur.

M. **The duration of the QRS complex.** Ventricular ectopy is usually associated with a QRS duration greater than 0.14 sec (Wellens and associates, 1978[13]) (See Figs. 232 to 235). Conversely, a QRS duration of 0.14 sec or less, strongly favours aberrant ventricular conduction[13] (see Fig. 236).

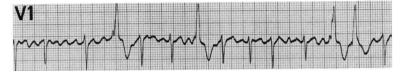

Fig. 236. The electrocardiogram (lead V1) reflects atrial fibrillation as evidenced by the irregular baseline due to distortion by the fibrillatory waves, and the irregular ventricular response. The bizarre QRS complexes are due to aberrant ventricular conduction, as is evident from the following: A. The initial vector is the same as that associated with the normally conducted beats. B. There is no attempt at a compensatory pause.

4. The presence or absence of an attempt at a compensatory pause in atrial fibrillation

When phasic aberrant ventricular conduction complicates atrial fibrillation, the bizarre QRS complex of the aberration is not usually nor necessarily followed by a compensatory pause, or an attempt at a compensatory pause (Fig. 236). When, however, a ventricular extrasystole, for example, complicates atrial fibrillation, the bizarre QRS complex is usually followed by a long or relatively long pause. This is due to concealed retrograde conduction of the extrasystolic impulse into the A-V node, thereby rendering it refractory to the immediately ensuing fibrillation impulses.

ATRIAL FLUTTER WITH ABERRANT VENTRICULAR CONDUCTION SIMULATING EXTRASYSTOLIC VENTRICULAR BIGEMINY

Phasic aberrant ventricular conduction is particularly prone to occur during atrial flutter, when relatively early conducted beats may be conducted with aberration, and may consequently mimic extrasystolic ventricular rhythm.

MECHANISM

The manifestation of aberrant ventricular conduction during atrial flutter is basically due to the presence of alternating 4:1 and 2:1 atrioventricular (A-V) block. This will result in a form of ventricular bigeminal rhythm, since the 2:1 A-V block results in two beats which are inscribed in relatively quick succession, whereas the 4:1 A-V block results in a relatively long pause (Fig. 237). Furthermore, the conducted impulse terminating the 2:1 A-V block is relatively

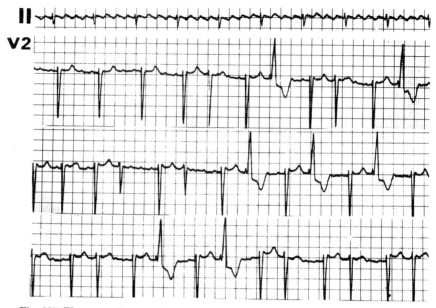

Fig. 237. Electrocardiogram showing atrial flutter with variable 4:1 and 2:1 A-V block. The impulses are conducted with normal intraventricular conduction and with aberration (see text).

premature and is, therefore, likely to be conducted with aberration. In addition, it is preceded by a long pause—the period of 4:1 A-V block. And since a long pause results in an ensuing prolongation of refractoriness, this too will favour the ensuing aberration.

The mechanism and principle are diagrammatically illustrated in Fig. 238. Impulses 1 to 11 represent flutter impulses. The conducted impulses—1, 5, 7, and 11—are also labelled a, b, c, and d. Beat c terminates the 2:1 episode of A-V block and is, therefore, relatively premature. It is consequently conducted with aberration. Furthermore, it is preceded by a relatively long ventricular cycle—the preceding period of 4:1 A-V conduction. This favours an ensuing prolongation of refractoriness. The second beat of the bigeminal couplet is consequently conducted with aberration and mimics extrasystolic ventricular bigeminy. This manifestation is illustrated in Fig. 237.

The electrocardiogram (a strip of Standard lead II, and a continuous strip of lead V2) was recorded from a 40-year-old man with congestive cardiac failure due to a congestive cardiomyopathy. He was not on digitalis therapy.

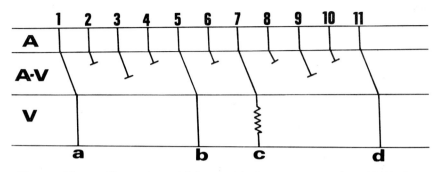

Fig. 238. Diagram illustrating atrial flutter with alternating 4:1 and 2:1 A-V block. The conducted impulse beginning a 4:1 conduction sequence is conducted with aberration.

Standard lead II shows atrial flutter with 4:1 A-V block. Lead V2 shows the following:

1. Periods of uncomplicated 4:1 A-V block—the first four beats of the tracing.

2. A period of 4:1 A-V block alternating with 2:1 A-V block, and associated with normal intraventricular conduction—the last six beats of the bottom strip.

3. The second half of the middle strip reflects three bizarre QRS complexes alternating with normal QRS complexes. This simulates extrasystolic ventricular bigeminy. Analysis, however, reveals that these are most likely to be aberrantly conducted flutter impulses which terminate cycles of 2:1 A-V conduction. This is evident from the following characteristics of the aberration:

(*a*) The initial QRS vector of the abnormal QRS complex is the same as that of the normally conducted QRS complex.

(*b*) The QRS complex has a triphasic configuration.[7]

(*c*) Beats 4 and 6 of the middle strip show lesser degrees of aberration.

(*d*) The pause following the bizarre beat is identical to the pause created by the 4:1 A-V conduction with normal intraventricular conduction.

Comment

The accurate differentiation of phasic aberrant ventricular conduction from ventricular ectopic conduction is of particular importance in the context of atrial flutter, since the diagnosis of aberration would be an indication to begin or increase the digitalis therapy, whereas the diagnosis of extrasystolic ventricular bigeminy would be an indication to stop digitalis therapy, or to proceed with caution.

REFERENCES

1 GOUAUX J. L. & ASHMAN R. (1947) Auricular fibrillation with aberration simulating ventricular paroxysmal tachycardia. *Am. Heart J.* **34**, 366.

2 LEWIS T. (1912) Observations upon disorders of the heart's action. *Heart* **3**, 279.

3 LEWIS T., DRURY A. N. & BULGER H. A. (1921) Observations upon flutter and fibrillation. Part VI. *Heart* **8**, 83.

4 MARRIOTT H. J. L. (1972) *Practical Electrocardiography*, 4th Edition. Baltimore: Williams and Wilkins Co.

5 MARRIOTT H. J. L. (1972) *Workshop in Electrocardiography*. Oldmar, Florida: Tampa Tracings.

6 MARRIOTT H. J. L. & FOGG E. (1970) Constant monitoring for cardiac dysrrhythmia and blocks. *Mod. Conc. Cardiovasc. Dis.* **39**, 103.

7 MINES G. R. (1913) On dynamic equilibrium in the heart. *J. Physiol. (Lond.)* **46**, 349.

8 SANDLER A. & MARRIOTT H. J. L. (1965) The differential morphology of anomalous ventricular complexes of right bundle branch block-type in Lead V1. Ventricular ectopic versus aberration. *Circulation* **31**, 551.

9 SCHAMROTH L. & CHESLER E. (1963) Phasic aberrant ventricular conduction. *Brit. Heart J.* **25**, 219.

10 SHEARN M. A. & RYTAND D. A. (1953) Intermittent bundle branch block: observations with special reference to the critical heart rate. *Arch. intern. Med.* **91**, 440.

11 TRENDELENBURG W. (1903) Ueber den Wegfall der Compensatorischen Ruhe am spontan Schlagenden/Froschherzen. *Arch. Anat. Physiol. (Lps.) Physiol. Abt.* 311.

12 VESELL H. (1941) Critical rate in ventricular conduction: unstable bundle branch block. *Amer. J. med. Sci.* **202**, 198.

13 WELLENS H. J. J., BAR F. W. & LIE K. I. (1978) The value of the electrocardiogram in the differential diagnosis of a tachycardia with a widened QRS complex. *Am. J. Medicine* **64**, 27.

SECTION 5
CORRELATIVE ESSAY

Structural Nodal Disease:
The So-called Sick Sinus Syndrome

Chapter 26
Structural Nodal Disease: the So-called Sick Sinus Syndrome

NOMENCLATURE

The term 'Sick Sinus Syndrome' was used by Lown (1967)[5] and later by Ferrer in 1968[1] to connote an inherent abnormality of the sino-atrial node. The condition has also been called the 'Sluggish Sinus Syndrome'[12, 17] and the 'Lazy Sinus Syndrome'.[3] These terms, while alliterative, 'catchy' and conveniently descriptive are perhaps not sufficiently comprehensive. For, as will become abundantly clear, it is not only the S-A node which is 'sick' but also the A-V node and its appendages, and possibly other pacemaking centres as well. The involvement of the S-A node as well as the A-V node and possibly other parts of the conducting system has also been termed a 'panconduction defect' by Rasmussen (1971),[11] although it will also become evident that the condition is not only associated with disordered impulse conduction, but also disordered impulse formation. 'Double Nodal Disease' as it is termed by Marriott (1972)[7] is more definitive. 'Structural Nodal Disease' (Schamroth, 1980)[16] would appear to be a most suitable title since it embraces disease of both the S-A and A-V nodes and their appendages, and clearly separates diseases due to structural change from metabolic and pharmacologic abnormalities.

ELECTROCARDIOGRAPHIC MANIFESTATIONS

Structural nodal disease manifests with abnormalities of impulse formation and impulse conduction involving the S-A node and the

279

A-V node and its appendages: the bundle of His, the bundle branches and the fascicles of the left bundle branch. Basically, the manifestation is one of intermittent or sustained atrial bradycardia which may be due to sinus bradycardia, S-A block or sinus arrest. This is usually associated with: (*a*) conduction defects in the A-V node and its appendages, (*b*) poor or inadequate escape rhythm, and (*c*) a possible complicating supraventricular tachyarrhythmia. The syndrome may thus present with a wide potential spectrum of disordered rhythms, some of which are presented in outline below.

1. *Sinus bradycardia*

The syndrome may manifest with sinus bradycardia which is not due to such obvious non-structural causes as digitalis administration, beta blockade, quinidine, procainamide, uraemia, obstructive jaundice, myxoedema, and a vagotonic athletic constitution. The sinus bradycardia is reflected by a sinus rate of less than 50 to 60 per minute in the adult which may be persistent or episodic. The sinus bradycardia of structural nodal disease rarely manifests as an isolated abnormality.

2. *Marked sinus arrhythmia*

The sinus bradycardia may be associated with marked sinus arrhythmia.

3. *Inadequate sinus tachycardia*

The syndrome may also be suspected when an expected sinus tachycardia is inadequate or fails to materialize in cases of fever, pain or congestive cardiac failure. The diagnosis may also be considered when the sinus rate fails to accelerate with exercise, or the administration of vagolytic drugs such as atropine.

4. *Uncomplicated escape rhythm secondary to marked S-A depression*

The syndrome may be suspected when a slow idionodal or idioventricular escape rhythm controls the activation of the entire heart. For example, the cardiac rhythm may manifest as an idionodal escape rhythm at a rate of 40 to 60 beats per minute with anterograde activation of the ventricles and retrograde activation of the atria. It is then clear that (*a*) the potential sinus rate must be below 40 to 60 beats per minute, or (*b*) there is sinus arrest or (*c*) there is complete S-A block, for otherwise the sinus rhythm would manifest.

5. *Sinus bradycardia with A-V block*

The sinus bradycardia of structural nodal disease may be associated with first-, second- or third-degree A-V block. The A-V block may be manifest, or may only be revealed, for example, by atrial pacing. It is present in about two-thirds of the cases of sinus bradycardia due to structural nodal disease (Narula 1971;[9] Rosen and associates 1971;[14] Rubenstein and associates 1971[15]).

6. *Sinus bradycardia or second-degree S-A block with escape rhythm*

The sinus bradycardia or second-degree S-A block of structural nodal disease may lead to escape rhythm—usually an idionodal escape rhythm. The escape rhythm may co-exist with the electrocardiographic manifestations of sinus bradycardia or second-degree S-A block, thereby leading to complex interplay of the sinus and escape rhythms. If, however, the sinus bradycardia or the S-A block is profound, the escape rhythm may be in complete control of cardiac activation and thus present as an uncomplicated escape rhythm (as discussed in section 4 above).

7. *Normal sinus rhythm or sinus bradycardia with S-A and A-V block, and failure of escape rhythm*

Structural nodal disease may manifest with second-degree S-A block which may be of the Type I (an S-A Wenckebach conduction) or Type II. The S-A block may occur in association with normal sinus rhythm or sinus bradycardia. The second-degree S-A block of structural nodal disease may, and usually does, manifest with concomitant first-, second- or third-degree A-V block. The long periods occasioned by the blocked sinus impulses are usually associated with a failure of escape rhythm to supervene.

8. *Profound sinus bradycardia, S-A block or sinus arrest with or without A-V block and with failure of, or inadequate, escape rhythm*

Adequate escape rhythm may fail to develop with marked sino-atrial depression. When this occurs the patient may experience frequent attacks of vertigo and syncope.

9. *Atrial fibrillation or atrial flutter with slow ventricular response*

Structural nodal disease may be suspected when atrial fibrillation or atrial flutter is associated with a slow or relatively slow ventricular response, and digitalis, verapamil or beta blockade, can be ruled out as a causal factor.

10. *Failure to resume sinus rhythm after cardioversion for atrial flutter or fibrillation*

When normal or adequate sinus rhythm fails to resume after cardioversion for atrial flutter or fibrillation, the possibility of structural nodal disease should be considered. The flutter or fibrillation may, under such a circumstance, be the end result of the bradycardia–tachycardia syndrome (see section 15 below).

11. *Prolonged return cycle following premature discharge of the S-A pacemaker*

When the sino-atrial pacemaker is prematurely discharged, for example, by an atrial extrasystole or a retrogradely conducted A-V nodal or ventricular extrasystole, it tends to be momentarily depressed. This will lead to a relatively long return cycle. This return cycle may be inordinately long in structural nodal disease and is usually pathological when it exceeds the basic sinus cycle by 25 per cent.[2, 6]

12. *Intra-atrial block*

The existence of atrial disease may be suspected when the electrocardiogram manifests with abnormally wide and/or deformed P waves.

13. *Changing P wave vectors—atrial escape*

The structural nodal disease may manifest with changing P wave shape and changing orientation of the P wave vector. This reflects an atrial escape rhythm secondary to sinus node depression. These atrial escape rhythms are seldom sustained, usually manifesting for short periods and, at times, for only one or two beats.

14. *Hemiblock*

The conducted beats associated with any of the aforementioned abnormal rhythms may be associated with a hemiblock, usually a left anterior hemiblock.

15. *The bradycardia–tachycardia syndrome*

The profound atrial slowing associated with the syndrome described above is not infrequently associated with paroxysmal supraventricular tachyarrhythmias: paroxysmal atrial flutter, fibrillation or tachycardia. These may first be manifest or precipitated after a long pause due to S-A block or sinus arrest. The diagnosis may be suspected when, following the termination of a paroxysm of atrial flutter, fibrillation or tachycardia, there is a period of exceptionally slow sinus bradycardia, which may be as slow as 25 to 35 beats per minute for a short period. The tachyarrhythmic manifestation may ultimately become established as a chronic, permanent atrial fibrillation.

The bradycardia–tachycardia syndrome thus represents an apparently paradoxical association of depressed conduction with hyperexcitability, the precise mechanism of which is not yet clear.

EVALUATION OF STRUCTURAL NODAL DISEASE

Evaluation of structural nodal disease is best considered with reference to sinus bradycardia. This is because sinus bradycardia is probably its simplest, commonest and earliest expression and, therefore, requires the most careful evaluation, especially if the patient is symmptomatic. The evaluation is based on:
  A. Clinical appraisal
  B. Prolonged monitoring
  C. Provocative tests

A. Clinical appraisal

Clinical appraisal must exclude such metabolic causes of sinus bradycardia as myxoedema and uraemia. And it is particularly important to exclude the drug effect of digitalis and beta receptor blockade.

B. Electrocardiographic monitoring

Structural nodal disease tends to pursue an unstable and capricious course, with irregular, alternating periods of normal and abnormal function. As a result, sinus bradycardia, sinus arrest, S-A block with the advent of escape rhythms or supraventricular tachyarrhythmias may not be manifest during physical examination. It consequently becomes necessary to institute long-term tape monitoring. This is especially so if the symptomatic episodes appear to be related to certain physical acts or other events. If, for example, profound bradycardia is expected during sleep it is mandatory to monitor during sleep.

C. Provocative tests

The presence of structural nodal disease may be revealed by certain provocative tests. These fall into two groups: (1) Vagolytic and sympathomimetic manoeuvres, and (2) overdrive suppression.

1. *Vagolytic and sympathomimetic manoeuvres*

The simplest of these is exercise. Failure of the sinus rate to accelerate with mild or moderate exercise would constitute a pointer to the presence of structural nodal disease. A possible vagal aetiology may also be excluded by the intravenous administration of 1–2 mg atropine sulphate which should increase the sinus rate to more than 90 impulses per minute.[14] Furthermore, atropine should also increase S-A nodal recovery time after overdrive suppression (see below). Stimulation of the S-A node by the intravenous administration of 1–2 mg isoproteranol in a suitable vehicle, should likewise increase the sinus rate to more than 90 per minute.

2. *Overdrive suppression*

This involves the assessment of sino-atrial recovery time after pacemaker suppression by a short period of rapid atrial pacing. Premature discharge of the S-A node, as occurs with atrial extrasystoles, atrial tachycardia or rapid atrial pacing, will momentarily suppress the inherent rhythmicity of the node so that the resumption of sinus rhythm is delayed. The compensatory pause following an atrial extrasystole, for example, is usually a little longer than the sinus cycle. This is because the extrasystolic impulse penetrates into

the S-A node and discharges it prematurely. This premature discharge depresses the S-A pacemaker momentarily so that it takes a
little longer than normal to reach maturity and fire spontaneously.
The same phenomenon occurs following spontaneous or paced atrial
tachycardia. The *recovery cycle* is also known as the *return cycle*, and
it is the assessment of this return cycle which constitutes the basis of
the overdrive suppression test, since the suppression will be more
marked in those pacemakers where automaticity is already impaired
by disease. Sino-atrial depression will also follow the introduction of
single electric stimuli to the atria—artificial atrial extrasystoles—
but a period of atrial pacing constitutes a better challenge to the S-A
node (Narula and associates, 1972[10]). A pacing rate of 120 beats per
minute for one to two minutes would appear to be ample in most
cases. The degree of sino-atrial suppression is related to the control
or basal sinus rate: the slower the resting rate the longer the
post-pacing pause (Mandel and associates, 1971[2,6]). The post-pacing
pause may be expressed as a percentage of the resting rate.[2,6] At
normal resting sinus rates of 60 to 80 beats per minute, the
post-pacing pause should not be more than 25 per cent of the resting
rate. While with sinus bradycardia at rates below 60 beats per
minute, the post-pacing pause should not be more than 20 per cent of
the resting rate (Narula and associates, 1972[10]). Values exceeding
these limits would suggest the presence of sino-atrial dysfunction. It
should be stressed that a single spontaneous atrial extrasystole with
a prolonged return cycle (as evaluated above) constitutes, at least, a
pointer to the presence of structural nodal disease or the so-called
sick sinus syndrome.

THE AETIOLOGY OF STRUCTURAL NODAL DISEASE

Structural nodal disease is basically due to a sclerodegenerative
process which has many causes, such as coronary artery disease,
including acute myocardial infarction, the cardiomyopathies, meta-
static disease,[8] primary muscular dystrophies, amyloid disease and
tuberosclerosis.[2] With adequate monitoring, structural nodal disease
has been estimated to occur in about 5 per cent of all cases of acute
myocardial infarction.[13] The manifestation is particularly prone with
occlusion of the left circumflex artery or the main right coronary
artery since either of these supplies the sino-atrial node with its
artery. Thus, sino-atrial dysfunction has been found in over half the
cases with acute inferior wall myocardial infarction (James, 1968).[4]
Conversely, it has been noted that when sino-atrial disease manifests

in acute myocardial infarction, almost all—31 of 32 cases—have inferior wall infarction (Rokseth and Hatle, 1971).[13]

CLINICAL PRESENTATION

Clinical manifestations range from the subtle to the profound. Subtle changes include irritability, and other minimal personality changes, which may result in errors of judgement. There may also be episodes of nocturnal wakefulness. Neurological deficits may manifest with transient pareses or slurring of speech. The patient may present with obvious and dramatic syncopal attacks. Periodic fulminating and unexplained episodes of acute pulmonary oedema have also been attributed to structural nodal disease (Ferrer, 1973).[2]

TREATMENT

Since structural nodal disease is due to a structural change within the S-A node and A-V node, the administration of atropine or isoproterenol is unlikely to be successful. The efficacy of these agents will, in any event, be determined by the provocative tests. Thus, in the majority of cases, the insertion of a demand pacemaker becomes necessary. And since associated disease of the A-V conduction system is not infrequent, pacing from the ventricles is indicated.

REFERENCES

1 FERRER M. I. (1968) The sick sinus syndrome in atrial disease. *JAMA* **206**, 645.
2 FERRER M. I. (1973) The sick sinus syndrome. *Circulation* **47**, 67.
3 GINKS W. R. (1970) Lazy sinus syndrome. *Proc. roy. Soc. Med.* **63**, 1307.
4 JAMES T. N. (1968) The coronary circulation and conduction system in acute myocardial infarction. *Prog. Cardiovasc. Dis.* **10**, 410.
5 LOWN B. (1967) Electrical reversion of cardiac arrhythmias. *Brit. Heart J.* **29**, 469.
6 MANDEL W., HAYAKAWA H., DANZIG R. & MARCUS H. S. (1971) Evaluation of sino-atrial node function in man by overdrive suppression. *Circulation* **44**, 59.
7 MARRIOTT H. J. L. (1972) *Workshop in Electrocardiography.* Tampa Tracings, Oldmar, Florida.
8 METZGER A. L., GOLDBERG A. N. & HUNTER R. L. (1971) Sick sinus node syndrome as the presenting manifestation of reticulum cell sarcoma. *Chest* **60**, 602.
9 NARULA O. S. (1971) Atrioventricular conduction defects in patients with sinus bradycardia. *Circulation* **44**, 1096.
10 NARULA O. S., SAMET P. & JAVIER R. P. (1972) Significance of the sinus-node recovery time. *Circulation* **45**, 140.
11 RASMUSSEN K. (1971) Chronic sinoatrial heart block. *Amer. Heart J.* **81**, 38.
12 REILLY A., ROSEN K., LOEB H., SINNO Z., RAHIMTOOLA S. H. & GUNNAR R. (1970)

Cardiac conduction in the 'sluggish sinus node' syndrome. *Circulation* **42** (suppl. III), 42.

13 ROKSETH R. & HATLE L. (1971) Sinus arrest in acute myocardial infarction. *Brit. Heart J.* **33**, 639.

14 ROSEN K. M., LOEB H. S., SINNO Z., RAHIMTOOLA S. H. & GUNNAR R. M. (1971) Cardiac conduction in patients with symptomatic sinus node disease. *Circulation* **43**, 836.

15 RUBENSTEIN J. J., SCHULMAN CH. L., YURCHAK P. M. & DE SANCTIS R. W. (1972) Clinical spectrum of the sick sinus syndrome. *Circulation* **46**, 5.

16 SCHAMROTH L. (1980) *Disorders of Cardiac Rhythm* (2nd edition). Blackwell Scientific Publications, Oxford, England.

17 TABATZNIK B., MOWRER M. M., SAMSON E. B. & PREMPREE A. (1969) Syncope in the 'sluggish sinus node syndrome'. *Circulation* **40** (suppl. III), 200.

Chapter 27
General Considerations and Correlative Observations

THE APPROACH TO ELECTROCARDIOGRAPHIC INTERPRETATION

For adequate electrocardiographic interpretation it is clearly essential to examine every part and aspect of the recording; but perhaps even as important is the necessity to seek out actively the possible abnormal patterns. It is, therefore, desirable to approach the interpretation of electrocardiograms with specific objectives in mind. The following scheme, while by no means complete, lists some of the important correlative features and abnormal patterns which must be purposefully and specifically looked for in electrocardiographic interpretation.

THE P WAVE

(*a*) *Atrial enlargement.* The diagnosis of atrial enlargement is usually best made from the P wave pattern in Standard lead II or, in the case of left axis deviation of the P wave, in Standard lead I; and lead V1.

(*b*) *Inverted P waves in Standard leads II and III and lead AVF* suggest retrograde activation of the atria. This may occur with impulses arising within or passing through the A-V node, and with retrograde Kent bundle conduction.

(*c*) *Inverted P waves in Standard lead I* suggests:
    (i) Incorrect electrode placement (right arm lead attached to left arm, and vice versa).
    (ii) Mirror-image dextrocardia.
    (iii) Possible retrograde atrial activation from an impulse conducted through a left-sided bundle of Kent.

THE P–R INTERVAL

(*a*) A *prolonged P–R interval* suggests:
    (i) Coronary artery disease   or (ii) Digitalis effect.

(*b*) A *short P–R interval* may be due to:
    (i) A dissociated beat.   (iii) A-V nodal rhythm.
    (ii) The W-P-W syndrome.

THE QRS COMPLEX

(*a*) The diagnosis of *inferior wall myocardial infarction* is made from the typical infarction pattern—pathological Q wave, raised S-T segment and inverted T wave—in *Standard leads II and III, and lead AVF*; leads orientated to the inferior or diaphragmatic surface of the heart.

(*b*) The diagnosis of *anterior wall myocardial infarction* is made from the typical pattern—pathological Q wave, raised S-T segment and inverted T wave in the *V leads, Standard lead I and lead AVL.*

(*c*) The diagnosis of *right bundle branch block* is usually made from the presence of an rSR′ or 'M'-shaped QRS complex in leads V1 and V2.

(*d*) The diagnosis of *left bundle branch* is usually made from the presence of a notched and widened 'M'-shaped QRS complex in leads V5 and V6.

(*e*) *Right ventricular hypertrophy* is usually suggested to tall R waves in leads V1 and V2 and right axis deviation.

(*f*) *Left ventricular hypertrophy* is usually suggested by tall R waves in leads V5 and V6 associated with deep S waves in leads V1 and V2. This may be associated with a 'strain' pattern: depressed convex-upward S-T segments in leads V5 and V6, and left atrial enlargement.

THE S-T SEGMENT

(*a*) *Coronary artery disease* is suggested by horizontality, plane depression or sagging of the S-T segment, particularly in Standard lead II and leads V5 and V6.

(*b*) *Digitalis effect* is suggested by a mirror-image correction mark shape of the S-T segment—usually seen in leads V5 and V6.

(*c*) *The 'strain pattern'*—depressed convex-upward S-T segment with inverted T wave—may be seen in leads V5 and V6 in left ventricular hypertrophy; and in leads V1 and V2 in right ventricular hypertrophy.

(*d*) *The hyperacute phase* of myocardial infarction and the variant form of angina pectoris (Prinzmetal's Angina) is reflected by slope-elevation of the S-T segment associated with a tall and widened T wave.

THE T WAVE

(*a*) Low or inverted T waves in most leads may be associated with coronary heart disease.

(*b*) Low or inverted T waves associated with generalized low voltage of the QRS complex suggest pericardial effusion or myxoedema.

(*c*) Tall peaked T waves in the precordial leads may be due to:

    (i) Acute subendocardial ischaemia or infarction.

    (ii) Recovering inferior infarction.

    (iii) Hyperkalaemia.

THE U WAVE

(*a*) An *inverted U wave* in Standard leads I and II, and leads V5 and V6 is usually due to:

    (i) coronary heart disease,

or

    (ii) hypertensive heart disease.

(*b*) A *prominent U wave* in the mid-precordial leads—(V3 to V5)—is commonly due to hypopotassaemia.

COMMON ASSOCIATIONS

Electrocardiographic Combinations	Suggested Diagnosis
1 Atrial fibrillation Right axis deviation	Mitral stenosis
2 'Left atrial' P wave Right axis deviation	Mitral stenosis

3 Atrial fibrillation
  Right axis deviation
  Left ventricular diastolic
    overload
	Mitral incompetence

4 *Very tall* 'right atrial' P waves
    in Standard lead II
  First degree A-V block
  Normal QRS axis
	Tricuspid stenosis

5 'Left atrial' P wave Left ventricular systolic overload	Hypertensive heart disease

The arrhythmias associated with hyperthyroidism

    Sinus tachycardia
    Atrial extrasystoles
    Paroxysmal atrial tachycardia
    Paroxysmal atrial flutter
    Paroxysmal atrial fibrillation
    Idionodal tachycardia
    Paroxysmal A-V nodal tachycardia

Note. Ventricular rhythms are not usually associated with hyperthyroidism, but may occur when there is associated cardiac decompensation.

SOME COMMON ELECTROCARDIOGRAPHIC MANIFESTATIONS OF CONGENITAL HEART DISEASE

Pulmonary stenosis

1. *P. congenitale.*
2. Right ventricular systolic overload: *very tall* R waves and S-T segment 'strain' pattern (depressed convex-upward S-T segments and inverted T waves) in leads orientated to the right ventricle—leads V1 to V3.
3. Right axis deviation.

The tetralogy of Fallot

As for pulmonary stenosis, but the T wave is usually inverted in lead V1 only, and usually upright (occasionally inverted) in leads V2 and V3 (Fig. 79).

Tricuspid atresia

    1.   Left axis deviation.
    2.   Left ventricular dominance.

Note. Most cases of cyanotic congenital heart disease manifest with right ventricular dominance and right axis deviation; tricuspid atresia is a notable exception.

Atrial septal defect

Ostium secundum type

      1. *Incomplete* or complete right bundle branch block.
      2. 1st degree A-V block.

Ostium primum type and *persistent A-V communis*

      1. Incomplete or complete right bundle branch block.
      2. *Left axis deviation* of the initial vector.

Ventricular septal defect with pulmonary hypertension (Fig. 239)

1. *Biventricular hypertrophy*

Right ventricular hypertrophy—right ventricular systolic overload.
Left ventricular hypertrophy—deep S waves over right precordial leads; tall R waves over left precordial leads.

    This results in large amplitude diphasic QRS complexes in many leads and is known as the *Katz-Wachtel Phenomenon.*

2. *Deep but narrow Q waves*

Deep but narrow Q waves (associated with tall R waves) over the left precordial leads—leads V5 and V6—are particularly suggestive of ventricular septal defect.

Patent ductus arteriosus

This condition is usually manifested by left ventricular diastolic overload.

Coarctation of the aorta

Left ventricular systolic overload.

Ebstein's anomaly

1. Tall peaked P waves in Standard lead II.
2. Right bundle branch block with small amplitude QRS complexes.
3. Wolff-Parkinson-White syndrome—Type B, i.e. the QRS complex

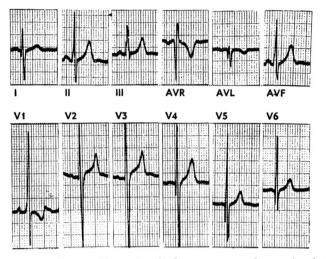

| I | II | III | AVR | AVL | AVF |

| V1 | V2 | V3 | V4 | V5 | V6 |

Fig. 239. Electrocardiogram illustrating the features commonly associated with ventricular septal defect. Note (*a*) evidence of right ventricular hypertrophy—tall R waves in leads V1 to V3; (*b*) evidence of left ventricular diastolic overload—tall R waves in leads V4 to V6, deep S waves in leads V2 and V3, *deep but narrow Q waves* in leads V4 to V6, and rather tall symmetrical T waves, and minimally elevated S-T segments, in leads V4 to V6; (*c*) the resultant large amplitude diphasic QRS complexes in Standard leads I, II, leads AVR, AVF and leads V2 to V5—the *Katz-Wachtel Phenomenon*. Note the small initial slur in lead V1.

is negative over the right precordial leads (Sodi-Pallares & Calder, 1956[1]).

4. Paroxysmal supraventricular tachycardia.

Corrected transposition of the great vessels

This condition is frequently associated with *A-V dissociation* due to high-grade A-V block. Thus, the combination of A-V dissociation and a pansystolic murmur in a young child is presumptive evidence of possible corrected transposition of the great vessels.

'Mirror-image' dextrocardia

1. Inverted P waves in Standard lead I (see also page 138).
2. All other deflections—QRS complex and T wave—are also negative in Standard lead I. This lead now resembles a normal lead AVR.

3. The normal appearances of Standard leads II and III are interchanged.

4. The QRS complexes are tallest in the right precordial leads—V1 and V2—and diminished progressively to the left.

Reversed arm electrodes

This will manifest as for mirror-image dextrocardia but the precordial lead complexes will be normal.

Anomalous left coronary artery

When the left coronary artery arises from the pulmonary artery the electrocardiogram reflects the patterns of *anterolateral infarction*, viz. pathological Q waves, raised and coved S-T segments, and inverted T waves in Standard lead I, lead AVL and the left precordial leads.

AN APPROACH TO THE DIAGNOSIS OF THE ARRHYTHMIAS

One of the more important aspects to the solution of an arrhythmia is the *behaviour of the P wave*. This is best seen in Standard lead II or lead VI; at times, special leads have to be used, viz. lead S5* or an oesophageal lead. The following procedure is recommended in the study of an arrhythmia.

1. Note the rate of the sinus discharge, i.e. the frequency of the P–P intervals. A rate exceeding 150 per minute in the adult usually, but not invariably, indicates a paroxysmal atrial tachycardia.

2. Note the rhythm or regularity of the P waves:

   (a) A *gradual* increase and diminution of the P–P intervals is characteristic of sinus arrhythmia.

   (b) A *sudden early P wave of different contour* denotes an atrial extrasystole. Note whether this is followed by a normal or aberrant QRS complex, or whether it is not followed by a QRS complex at all—a blocked atrial extrasystole.

3. If typical P waves cannot be identified, note whether the baseline has the 'saw-tooth' appearance of atrial flutter or the chaotic appearance of atrial fibrillation.

---

* The selector switch is set at S1; the right arm—negative—electrode is placed over the manubrium, and the left arm—positive—electrode is placed over the right fifth interspace adjacent to the sternum.

4. Note whether each P wave is followed by a QRS complex. If a P wave is not followed by a QRS complex, it may be due to (*a*) second-degree A-V block, in which case all the P–P intervals will be regular (allowing for possible sinus arrhythmia) or (*b*) a blocked atrial extrasystole, in which case the P wave related to the pause is premature and bizarre. Note that a blocked atrial extrasystole may be superimposed on the preceding T wave and consequently obscured; the situation may then mimic, and be mistaken for, S-A block. The T waves of all pauses must, therefore, be carefully scrutinized for deformity—no matter how slight.

Note the duration of the P–R interval. In the case of second-degree A-V block, note whether the dropped beat is preceded by a gradual lengthening of the P–R intervals—the Wenckebach Phenomenon.

5. Note whether the beat following a pause is a normal sinus beat or an atrial, A-V nodal, or ventricular, escape beat.

6. If the P waves are not related to the QRS complexes, A-V dissociation is present. This may be due to:

(*a*) *Paroxysmal ventricular tachycardia*: the QRS complexes will be bizarre and slightly irregular.

(*b*) *Non-paroxysmal or paroxysmal, nodal tachycardia*: the QRS complexes are usually normal in shape, or abnormal with the classic features of right or, less commonly, left bundle branch block. Dissociation may be incomplete in any of the above conditions: the rhythm is complicated by capture beats, i.e. interference-dissociation. This is characterized by a *sudden early beat* which is *related to a P wave.*

(*c*) *Complete A-V block*: The QRS complexes may be normal or bizarre and are usually recorded at a rate of less than 40 per minute.

7. An arrhythmia with a bizarre QRS pattern does not necessarily connote an ectopic ventricular origin, but may be due to *Phasic Aberrant Ventricular Conduction*; in such instances, the relationship of the P wave to the QRS complex and the contour of the QRS complex (particularly in lead V1 and the other precordial leads) will usually indicate the correct diagnosis.

Examples

(*a*) An early bizarre QRS complex during normal sinus rhythm may, at first glance, be mistaken for a ventricular extrasystole. If, however, it is preceded by a premature and abnormal P wave, it is due to an atrial extrasystole with phasic aberrant ventricular conduction.

(*b*) A rapid rhythm characterized by repeated bizarre QRS complexes may be due to:

(i) Supraventricular tachycardia with phasic aberrant ventricular conduction: *all* the bizarre QRS complexes will be preceded by P waves.

(ii) Paroxysmal ventricular tachycardia. The bizarre QRS complexes may be completely dissociated from the P waves (the rhythm may also be complicated by possible capture beats). When the ectopic ventricular impulses are conducted retrogradely to the atria, each QRS complex will be related to an ensuing P wave. When the QRS:P relationship cannot be established with certainty, the contour of the QRS complex in the precordial leads, particularly lead V1 (or MCL1), may indicate the correct diagnosis (see Chapter 25, page 269).

SOME FURTHER OBSERVATIONS ON ABNORMAL RHYTHMS

A SLOW REGULAR VENTRICULAR RHYTHM may be due to:
1. Sinus bradycardia
2. Complete A-V block with idioventricular rhythm
3. Normal sinus rhythm with 2:1 A-V block
4. Normal sinus rhythm with 2:1 S-A block (very rare)
5. Atrial flutter with high-grade 4:1 A-V block
6. Sinus default with idionodal escape rhythm
7. Sinus default with idioventricular escape rhythm.

CAUSES OF IRREGULAR VENTRICULAR RHYTHM

1. Atrial fibrillation
2. Frequent and irregularly occurring atrial and/or ventricular extrasystoles
3. Atrial flutter with second-degree A-V block and varying A-V conduction ratios
4. Paroxysmal atrial tachycardia with varying second-degree A-V block
5. *Marked* respiratory sinus arrhythmia.

'SLOW' ATRIAL FIBRILLATION

'Slow' atrial fibrillation usually reflects treatment with digitalis; or, in the absence of digitalis therapy, structural nodal disease—the so-called Sick Sinus Syndrome. A more correct description is—atrial fibrillation with slow or diminished ventricular response.

SOME COMMON CAUSES OF BIGEMINAL RHYTHM

Alternate ventricular extrasystoles (common)
Alternate atrial or nodal extrasystoles
Any form of 3:2 A-V block
Atrial flutter with alternating 4:1 and 2:1 A-V block.

ABSENT P WAVES

Absent P waves may be due to:
1. S-A block
2. Atrial fibrillation
3. Hyperkalaemia
4. A-V nodal rhythm (the P waves may be hidden within the QRS complexes).

A LONG PAUSE interrupting regular rhythm may be caused by:
1. A 'dropped beat' as a result of second-degree A-V block
2. A 'dropped beat' as a result of S-A block
3. A blocked or non-conducted atrial extrasystole.

When the P–R INTERVAL BECOMES PROGRESSIVELY SHORTER, A-V DISSOCIATION is usually present.

EXTRASYSTOLES occur PREMATURELY; ESCAPE BEATS occur LATE.

PAROXYSMAL ATRIAL RHYTHM (tachycardia, paroxysmal or flutter fibrillation) in a young person without obvious evidence of cardiac disease raises the possibility of:
1. Thyrotoxicosis
2. The W-P-W syndrome
3. Lone atrial fibrillation.

FURTHER CORRELATIVE OBSERVATIONS

TALL SYMMETRICAL T WAVES IN THE PRECORDIAL LEADS

These may be due to:
1. Acute subendocardial ischaemia, injury or infarction
2. Recovering inferior wall myocardial infarction

3. Hyperacute phase of anterior wall myocardial infarction
4. Prinzmetal's angina
5. True posterior wall myocardial infarction
6. Hyperkalaemia.

GENERALIZED LOW VOLTAGE

This may be due to:
1. Incorrect standardization
2. Emphysema
3. Obesity or thick chest wall
4. Pericardial effusion or constrictive pericarditis
5. Myxoedema
6. Hypopituitarism.

ACUTE RHEUMATIC FEVER

This is frequently associated with:
1. Sinus tachycardia
2. Non-paroxysmal A-V nodal tachycardia—idionodal tachy-cardia
3. Prolonged P–R interval
4. Second-degree A-V block
5. Prolonged Q–T interval.

THE TRANSITION ZONE

The precordial transition zone characterizes the transition from the rS complexes, recorded by leads orientated to the right ventricle, to the qR complexes, recorded by leads orientated to the left ventricle. This zone is usually reflected by lead V3 or lead V4. The complexes in these leads are usually intermediate in shape between the typical rS and qR configurations, and the T waves may be notched or bifid. This zone is therefore, characterized by atypical or even bizarre deflections and caution should be exercised in interpreting abnormality solely from these leads.

Electrocardiographic abnormalities may occur in normal healthy persons and in the absence of organic heart disease.

Organic heart disease may occur with normal electrocardiographic patterns.

Serial electrocardiographic studies are of particular value, as a changing pattern is usually significant.

Inquiry should always be made whether the patient has been taking drugs. Digitalis is the arch-simulator and may mimic almost any abnormal electrocardiographic pattern.

The electrocardiogram is only a supplementary aid to diagnosis and must always be used by the clinician in conjunction with the clinical examination.

REFERENCE

1 SODI-PALLARES D. & CALDER R. M. (1956) *New Bases of Electrocardiography.* St. Louis: C. V. Mosby and Co.

STANDARDIZATION OF THE ELECTROCARDIOGRAPH

The electrocardiograph must be correctly standardized before each recording. Incorrect standardization reflects incorrect mechanical operation of the electrocardiograph and will distort the electrocardiographic deflections.

Correct normal standardization

Correct normal technical standardization is represented in Diagrams A of Fig. 240. Normal conventional standardization is 1 mV. This will result in a standardization signal which is 1 cm—2 large squares—in amplitude. Furthermore, if the recording stylus has a correct pressure on the recording edge, the corners of the standardization signal will be at right-angles to each other.

Overdamping

Overdamping is incorrect technical standardization due to excessive pressure of the recording stylus on the recording edge. The excursions of the recording stylus are, therefore, somewhat impeded and will become lesser in amplitude. The effects are illustrated in Diagram B of Fig. 240. The standardization signal will reflect a slurring of the upstroke with the upper horizontal line, and also a slurring of the downstroke with the baseline. All the electrocardiographic deflections will be smaller in amplitude, and a terminal S wave, for example, may, in fact, disappear completely.

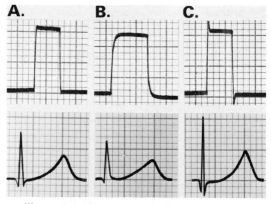

Fig. 240. Diagrams illustrating: (A) correct normal standardization, (B) overdamping and (C) underdamping—'overshoot'.

Underdamping: 'overshoot'

'Overshoot' is the expression of incorrect technical standardization as a result of too little pressure of the recording stylus on the recording edge. The excursions of the stylus are thus relatively unimpeded. The movement of the stylus is more free and the excursions are, therefore, greater in amplitude. The effects are illustrated in Diagrams C of Fig. 240. The standardization signal will reflect a sharply pointed 'overshoot' on both upstroke and the downstroke. All the electrocardiographic deflections may consequently be increased in amplitude and exaggerated. Furthermore, a terminal S wave may become exaggerated, or an S wave may, in fact, appear when it should normally be absent.

FORM FOR ROUTINE REPORTING

Name: ....   Date: ....

Age: ....   Registration No.: ....

Drugs: ....   Ward and Bed No.: ....

....

Rate: e.g. 140 per minute

Rhythm: e.g. sinus and arrhythmia

P wave: e.g. tall and peaked in Standard lead II and
                      lead V1

P–R interval: e.g. 0.26 second

QRS complex:

    Width ....   e.g. 0.12 second in lead V1

    Axis ....   e.g. $-30°$

    Configuration ....   e.g. normal
                      or
                      deep Q waves in leads ....
                      or
                      R–R complex in leads ....
                      or
                      deep S waves in leads ....

S-T segment: e.g. coved
                      raised   } in leads ....
                      plane depression

T wave: low to inverted throughout
                      or
                      tall and symmetrical in leads ....

U wave: e.g. inverted in leads ....
                      or
                      prominent in leads ....

Comments: List abnormalities here

1.   e.g. 1. *P. mitrale*

2.   2. first-degree A-V block

3.   3. right axis deviation

4.   4. right ventricular systolic overload
                      or

5.   e.g. 1. atrial fibrillation

6.   2. right bundle branch block

Conclusions: *Suggested terminology:*
                    1. Normal electrocardiogram.
                    2. The electrocardiogram is within nor-
                    mal limits.

3. Borderline electrocardiogram (list questionable features).

4. Abnormal electrocardiogram characteristic (or diagnostic) of ....

5. Abnormal electrocardiogram suggestive of ....

6. Abnormal electrocardiogram consistent with ....

7. Abnormal non-specific electrocardiogram (list abnormal features).

Additional remarks:

1. Suggest serial records.

2. Suggest additional leads.

3. Record Standard lead III in deep inspiration and deep expiration.

4. Suggest exercise test.

Appendix

ELECTROCARDIOGRAPHIC MEASUREMENTS
(Fig. 241)

1.   The **P–R interval** is measured from the *beginning* of the P wave to the *beginning* of the QRS complex irrespective of whether the QRS complex begins with a Q or an R wave.

2.   The **Q–T interval** is measured from the *beginning* of the QRS complex to the *end* of the T wave.

3.   The **intrinsicoid deflection** begins after the maximum QRS deflection has been inscribed, i.e. at the *peak of the R wave in qR complexes*, and at the *lowest point of the S wave in rS complexes*.

4.   The **ventricular activation time**—**VAT**—is the interval between the beginning of the QRS complex and the onset of the intrinsicoid deflection.

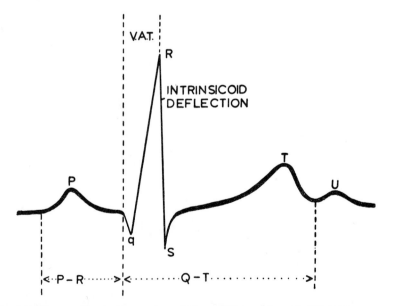

Fig. 241. Diagram illustrating various electrocardiographic measurements.

303

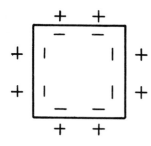

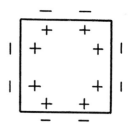

Fig. 242. Diagram illustrating a polarized or resting cell.

Fig. 243. Diagram illustrating a depolarized or activated cell.

ELEMENTARY ELECTROPHYSIOLOGY

In a healthy resting muscle cell, certain molecules dissociate into positive and negative ions. The positively charged ions are on the outer surface, and the negatively charged ions on the inner surface, of the cell membrane (Figs. 242 and 244). The positive charges are exactly equal in number to the negative charges. When this occurs the cell is in a state of electrical balance and is said to be **polarized.**

Note: When two electrical charges of equal and opposite direction, i.e. one positive ion and one negative ion, are juxtaposed on either side of a membrane, they constitute a **Dipole** (Fig. 245).

When two charged ions of equal and opposite direction are situated *next to each other on the surface of an excitable tissue*, they constitute a **Doublet** (Fig. 245). The term 'doublet' was introduced by Craib (1927)[1] to distinguish it from the dipole.

When the cell is *stimulated* or *injured*, the negative ions migrate to the outer surface of the cell and the positive charges pass into the cell, i.e. the polarity is reversed. This process is termed depolarization (Figs. 243 and 245). With recovery, positive charges return to the outer surface and negative charges migrate into the cell. This process is termed repolarization, i.e. the polarity or electrical balance of the cell is re-established.

﹒A series of cells in the resting state will all have positive surface charges. There is consequently no difference in surface electrical potential, and no current flows (Fig. 244).

If a stimulus travels through these resting (polarized) cells, those cells initially activated or depolarized will have negative surface charges whilst those not yet activated will have positive surface charges (Fig. 245). A potential electrical difference will therefore

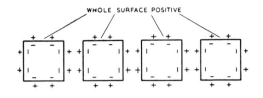

Fig. 244. Diagram illustrating polarized or resting cardiac muscle. All cells have positive surface charges.

exist between the *surface* of the excitable cells and the *surface* of the adjacent resting cells and a current will flow, i.e. the surface boundary between excitable and non-excitable tissue is characterized by a doublet. And as a doublet will always exist between the surfaces of excited and resting cells, *the flow of an electrical current may be viewed as a series of doublets* (Craib, 1927[1]).

This current will have a positive 'head' and a negative 'tail'. A unipolar electrode, or positive pole of a bipolar electrode, orientated towards the oncoming 'head' will record a positive or upward deflection; a unipolar electrode, or negative pole of a bipolar electrode, orientated towards the receding 'tail' will record a negative or downward deflection (Fig. 1).

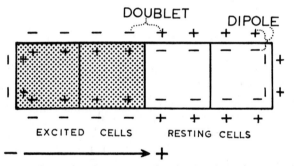

Fig. 245. Diagram illustrating the passage of excitation through a potentially excitable tissue. Note (*a*) excited cells—shaded area; the surface is electrically negative; (*b*) resting cells—the surface is electrically positive; (*c*) a *Dipole*—a pair of opposite charges on either side of the cell membrane; (*d*) a *Doublet*—a pair of adjacent but opposite charges on the surface of the membrane.

THE CURRENT OF INJURY

Injured myocardial tissue is reflected by a raised S-T segment in leads orientated to the injured surface, and by a depressed S-T segment in leads orientated to the uninjured surface. The mechanism governing this manifestation has not, as yet, been fully elucidated. One of the postulates is presented below.

Mechanism

Resting healthy myocardium has an electrically positive surface charge. When the whole muscle is in a resting state, all the surface charges are positive, no difference of electrical potential exists on the surface, and there is therefore no flow of current (Fig. 246A).

When heart muscle is either *stimulated* or *injured* its surface becomes electrically negative (see page 304, Fig. 245). If only part of the muscle strip is injured (Figs. 246B and 252), the injured part will

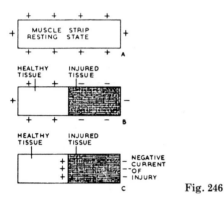

Fig. 246

have a negative surface charge and the adjacent healthy muscle will have a positive surface charge. This surface difference in potential between the injured and uninjured tissues leads to a flow of current. (See also Craib's 'doublet concept'—page 305). Thus, in effect, when a portion of heart muscle is injured, a continuous negative current— the current of injury—is emitted from the injured surface while a continuous positive current is emitted from the side of the injured tissue adjacent to the healthy muscle (Figs. 246C and 252A).

When the ventricle is injured as a result of myocardial infarction, a layer of muscle immediately adjacent to the endocardial surface is usually spared (Figs. 247 to 251; see also Fig. 24).

Thus an infarct of the left ventricular wall which causes injury but not death of tissue will emit a continuous negative current to an

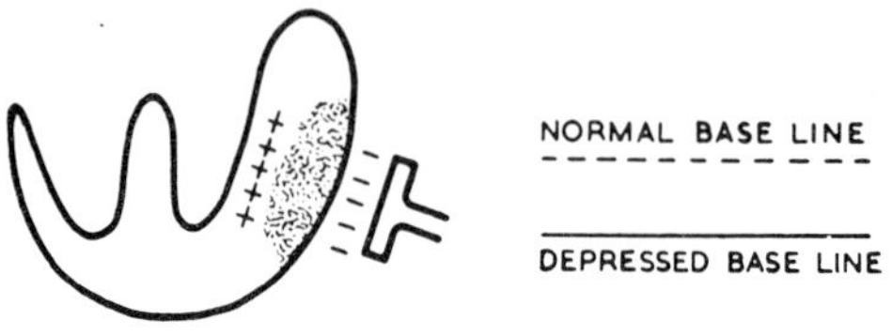

NORMAL BASE LINE

DEPRESSED BASE LINE

Fig. 247

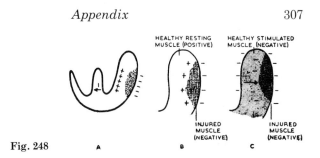

HEALTHY RESTING MUSCLE (POSITIVE)   HEALTHY STIMULATED MUSCLE (NEGATIVE)

INJURED MUSCLE (NEGATIVE)   INJURED MUSCLE (NEGATIVE)

Fig. 248   A   B   C

electrode orientated to the left ventricle, and this is recorded as a depressed baseline (Fig. 247). This is also illustrated in Fig. 252A where the baseline is depressed from position X to position Y.

Depolarization now occurs in the usual way from left to right through the interventricular septum (Fig. 248A), and then from right to left through the remaining healthy left ventricular wall (Fig. 248C).

As previously stated, *stimulation* of healthy muscle tissue will also result in a negative surface charge. Thus, after depolarization of the healthy part of the left ventricular wall, the healthy but stimulated tissue will also have a negative surface charge (Figs. 248C and 252B).

Since all surface charges have become electrically negative (i.e. of both the healthy stimulated tissue and the injured tissue), a potential difference no longer exists, no current flows and the continuous negative current of injury is abolished. As a result, the depressed baseline returns to the normal level giving the impression of a raised S-T segment (Figs. 249 and 252B). When the healthy stimulated muscle returns to the resting state, the negative current of injury reappears and the baseline is again depressed (Fig. 252C).

The myocardial injury is reflected by a **raised S-T segment in leads orientated to the injured surface.** The S-T is also **coved,** i.e. convex upwards (e.g. leads V2 to V6 in Fig. 30).

Conversely, an electrode facing the uninjured surface will record an elevated baseline due to the continuous emission of a positive current (Fig. 250).

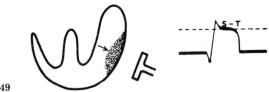

Fig. 249

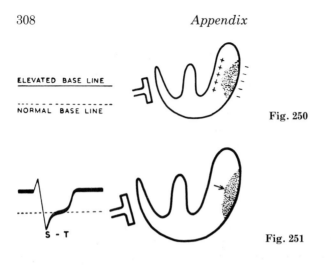

ELEVATED BASE LINE

NORMAL BASE LINE

Fig. 250

S - T

Fig. 251

During depolarization of the remaining healthy part of the left ventricle, the continuous positive force (directed to leads facing the uninjured surface) is abolished in a manner analogous to that described above. Consequently, the baseline momentarily returns to normal, giving the impression of a depressed S-T segment (e.g. lead AVL in Fig. 36).

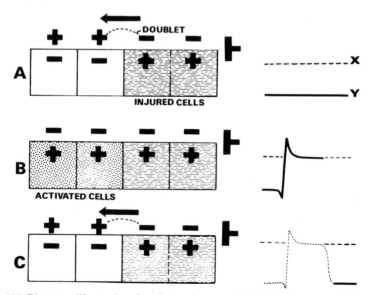

Fig. 252. Diagrams illustrating the effects of myocardial injury: the current injury.

THE TRANSMEMBRANE ACTION POTENTIAL

The electrocardiogram reflects the electrical activity of cardiac tissue. The electrical activity of a single muscle cell can be reflected experimentally by an intracellular micro-electrode which records the potential differences between it and an external reference electrode. The record is termed the **monophasic action potential** or the **transmembrane action potential.**

THE ACTION POTENTIAL OF A NON-PACEMAKING CELL

The resting potential of a myocardial cell is negative with respect to an external reference electrode and, by convention, is labelled phase 4 (Diagram A of Fig. 253). The resting potential of a non-pacemaking cell is stable, i.e. it remains at a constant, 'horizontal', negative, subthreshold level until depolarization by a propagated impulse results in its abrupt reversal, i.e. it becomes positive. The activated or excited state is termed the action potential (Diagram A of Fig. 253).

In common with all other types of excitable cells, the action potential of a non-pacemaking cardiac cell begins with an initial rapid depolarization—an abrupt upstroke which is labelled *Phase* 0 (Diagram A of Fig. 253). The action potential of cardiac cells differs from that of other excitable cells in exhibiting a slow delayed repolarization which may be divided into three phases:

Phase 1: a phase of early and rapid repolarization.

Phase 2: a phase of slow repolarization—termed *the plateau.*

Phase 3: a terminal phase of relatively rapid repolarization.

During the terminal phase of depolarization (Phase 0), as well as

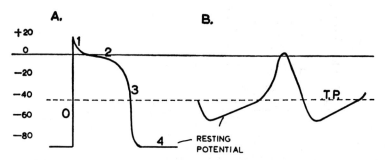

Fig. 253. Diagram illustrating A. Action potential of a non-pacemaking cell, and B. Action potential of a pacemaking cell.

during the early stages of repolarization (Phase 1 and the early part of Phase 2), the inside of the cell becomes temporarily positive in relation to the outside. This is termed the *overshoot* or *reversal*, and is represented in Diagram A of Fig. 253 by that part of the action potential which is situated above the zero level.

THE ACTION POTENTIAL OF A PACEMAKING CELL

The action potential of a pacemaking cell differs from that of a non-pacemaking cell in several respects (Diagram B of Fig. 253). The velocity of the upstroke of Phase 0 is somewhat slower. The reversal is small or absent. The peak is rounded. Phase 2 has a steeper decline and, therefore, does not usually exhibit the characteristic plateau configuration. The magnitude—or 'depth'—of the resting potential is less than that found with non-pacemaking cells. The most characteristic feature of a pacemaking cell, however, and its most striking difference from a non-pacemaking cell, is the presence of **slow spontaneous depolarization during Phase 4—diastolic depolarization.** The record reveals a 'resting' potential that exhibits a gradual upward slope. This slow diastolic depolarization begins immediately after Phase 3 resulting in a gradual loss of resting potential, i.e. the resting potential becomes less negative; and when the resting potential is reduced to a critical threshold level, there is a *smooth* but rapid transition to the upstroke of Phase 0 (Draper & Weidemann, 1951[2]).

The effect of diastolic depolarization is that the resting potential *regularly* and *automatically* reaches threshold level, thereby resulting in a regular, spontaneous, automatic discharge. Thus, diastolic depolarization reflects a pacemaking property—the property of automaticity or rhythmicity.

THE DERIVATION OF UNIPOLAR LEADS

The heart may be considered to lie in the centre of an equilateral triangle formed by the Standard leads (see Chapter 7 and Figs. 106 and 107). The apices of this triangle are thus, in a sense, the right arm, left arm and left leg electrodes (Fig. 254; see also Figs. 106 and 107). According to Einthoven, the sum of the potentials of these three leads is at any instant equal to zero. Thus, if these three leads are connected to a central terminal, the potential of this terminal will be zero (Fig. 254).

If this central terminal (also termed the neutral or indifferent

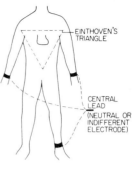

EINTHOVEN'S
TRIANGLE

CENTRAL
LEAD
(NEUTRAL OR
INDIFFERENT
ELECTRODE)

Fig. 254. Diagram illustrating the derivation of the neutral limb of a unipolar electrode. Note the three limb electrodes are joined to form a single lead—the neutral or indifferent lead.

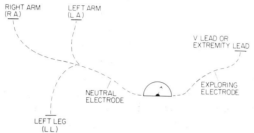

RIGHT ARM
(R A)

LEFT ARM
(L A)

V LEAD OR
EXTREMITY LEAD

NEUTRAL
ELECTRODE

EXPLORING
ELECTRODE

LEFT LEG
(L L)

Fig. 255. Diagram illustrating the derivation of a unipolar lead. The neutral limb is connected to the negative pole of the galvanometer; the exploring electrode is connected to the positive pole of the galvanometer.

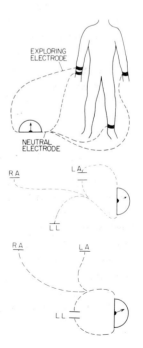

EXPLORING
ELECTRODE

NEUTRAL
ELECTRODE

Fig. 256. Diagram illustrating the derivation of lead VR. Note that the right arm has connections from both the neutral and exploring electrodes.

R A   L A

L L

Fig. 257. Diagram illustrating the derivation of lead VL. Note that the left arm has connections from both the neutral and exploring electrodes.

R A   L A

L L

Fig. 258. Diagram illustrating the derivation of lead VF. Note that the left leg has connections from both the neutral and exploring electrodes.

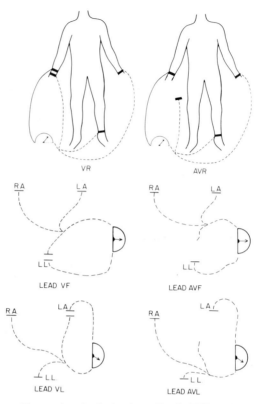

Fig. 259. Diagrams illustrating the derivation of leads AVR, AVL, and AVF.

electrode) is connected to one pole of the galvanometer, that lead will always have a potential value of zero. The electrode connected to the other pole of the galvanometer will record the true potential at any given point. This electrode is termed the exploring electrode (Fig. 255).

The development of this lead is due mainly to the work of Wilson and his associates (1944).[4]

EXTREMITY LEADS

Lead VR is obtained by connecting the exploring electrode to the right arm (Fig. 256).

Lead VL is obtained by connecting the exploring electrode to the left arm (Fig. 257).

Lead VF is obtained by connecting the exploring electrode to the left leg (Fig. 258).

Using the above technique, the potential obtained by the exploring electrode is of low voltage. Goldberger (1942)[3] augmented this voltage by omitting the connection of the neutral terminal to the limb which is being tested and allowing it to hang free (Fig. 259). The addition of the letter A is used to designate the augmented lead.

REFERENCES

1 CRAIB W. H. (1927) A study of the electrical field surrounding heart muscle. *Heart* **14**, 71.

2 DRAPER M. H. & WEIDEMANN S. (1951) Cardiac resting action potentials recorded with an intracellular electrode. *J. Physiol. (Lond.)* **155**, 74.

3 GOLDBERGER E. (1942) A simple indifferent, electrocardiographic electrode of zero potential and a technique of obtaining augmented, unipolar, extremity leads. *Amer. Heart J.* **23**, 483.

4 WILSON F. N., JOHNSTON F. D., ROSENBAUM F., ERLANDER H., KOSSMAN C., HECHT H., COTRIM N., MENEZES DE OLIVEIRA R., SCARSI R. & BARKER P. S. (1944) The precordial electrocardiogram. *Amer. Heart J.* **27**, 19.

Index

Aberrant ventricular conduction   258
Aberration   258
Action potential, transmembrane   309
Activation of the ventricles   5
Acute cor pulmonale   85
Acute pulmonary embolism   87
Alternans electrical   140
Aneurysm, ventricular   40
Angina pectoris   45, 50
Anomalous left coronary artery   294
Anterior infarction   29
Anterolateral infarction   29, 30
Anterolateral peri-infarction block   132
Anteroseptal infarction   29, 87
Antidromic reciprocating
   tachycardia   232
Arrhythmias, classification of   149
Arrhythmias, diagnosis of   294
Ashman phenomenon   263
Asystole, ventricular   213
Atrial activation   105
  mode of   5
Atrial enlargement   102, 104, 288
Atrial extrasystoles   157
Atrial fibrillation   166
  'Lone'   168
  paroxysmal of W-P-W syndrome   238
Atrial flutter   168
  paraxoysmal of W-P-W syndrome   238
  with aberrant ventricular
    conduction   275
Atrial septal defect   292
Atrial tachycardia, extrasystolic,
   paroxysmal   163
Atrioventricular (A-V) block   207
  congenital   219
  first-degree   207
  high-grade   214
  Mobitz Type I   210
  Mobitz Type II   211
  second-degree   208
  third-degree   212
A-V by-pass   222
A-V dissociation   249
A-V nodal escape beat   245

A-V nodal extrasystoles   174
A-V nodal rhythms   171
  paroxysmal   175
A-V nodal tachycardia, extrasystolic,
   paroxysmal   175
A-V nodal tachycardia, idionodal   175
Axis deviation   114
Axis, electrical   106
Axis, lead   106
Axis, mean electrical   111

Bigeminal rhythm   297
Bigeminy, extrasystolic ventricular   185
Bigeminy, in atrial flutter   275, 297
Bigeminy, 'Rule of hair'   183
Block, arborization   79
Block, atrioventricular (A-V)   207
Block, peri-infarction   128
Block, sino-atrial (S-A)   205
Bradycardia–tachycardia
   syndrome   283
Bundle branch block   72
Bundle of Kent   222

Calcium effect   98
Capture beats   251
Chronic cor pulmonale   87
Clockwise rotation   15
Coarctation of the aorta   292
Compensatory pause   157, 183
Conducting system, anatomy of   147
Conducting system, physiology   147
Conduction ratio   209
Congenital A-V block   219
Congenital heart disease   291
Cor pulmonale, acute   85
Cor pulmonale, chronic   87
Coronary artery, anomalous   294
Coronary insufficiency   45
Corrected transposition of the great
   vessels   293
Counterclockwise rotation   15
Craib's concept   304

Current of injury   305

Delta wave   233
Depolarization, diastolic   310
Dextrocardia   36, 115, 138, 293
Diaphragmatic infarction   30
Diaphragmatic peri-infarction
      block   132
Diastolic depolarization   310
Diastolic overload   89
Digitalis   64, 126
      effect   93
      toxicity   94
Dipole   304
Dissociation, A-V   249
Doublet   304
Dual rhythms   151

Ebstein's anomaly   292
Einthoven Triangle   109
Einthoven, Willem   107
Electrical alternans   140
Electrical axis   106
Electrocardiograph,
      standardization   299
Electrocardiographic deflections,
      nomenclature of   6, 9
Emphysema   87, 116
Escape beat, A-V nodal   245
Escape rhythms   150, 244
Exercise test   57
   'Poor man's'   65
Extrasystoles, atrial   157
Extrasystoles, A-V nodal   174
Extrasystoles, interpolated
      ventricular   183
Extrasystoles, ventricular   179
Extrasystolic atrial tachycardia   163
Extrasystolic A-V nodal
      tachycardia   175
Extrasystolic ventricular bigeminy   185
Extrasystolic ventricular
      tachycardia   186, 188

Fibrillation, atrial   166
Fibrillation, ventricular   198
Flutter, atrial   168
Flutter-fibrillation   170
Flutter, ventricular   195
Fusion   268
Fusion beats   202
Fusion complexes, ventricular   255
Fusion, ventricular   191

Galvanometer, action of   3
'Giant T wave inversion'   213
Glaucoma   156
Goldberger lead   312

Heart block *see* Block, A-V
Heart, electrical field   106
Heart, rotation of   12
Heberden's angina   50
Hemiblock concept   117
Hexaxial reference system   110
Horizontal position   13
Hypercalcaemia   100
Hyperkalaemia   95
Hypertension   64
Hypertensive heart disease   290
Hypocalcaemia   98
Hypokalaemia   95
Hypothermia   139

Idionodal tachycardia   175
Idioventricular tachycardia   191
Infarction, anterior   29
Infarction, anterolateral   29, 30
Infarction, anteroseptal   29, 87
Infarction, diaphragmatic   36
Infarction, fully evolved phase of   19
Infarction, hyperacute phase of   24
Infarction, inferior   30, 87, 116
Infarction, localization of   28
Infarction, myocardial   19
Infarction, old   40
Infarction, posterior   30
Infarction, resolution   37
Infarction, subendocardial   43
Infarction, vector principles   128
Inferior infarction   30, 87, 116
Injury, current of   305
Injury, ischaemia   22
Injury, myocardial   21
Interference-dissociation   249, 250, 257
Interpolated ventricular
      extrasystoles   183
Intracardiac conduction,
      representation   15
Intrinsicoid deflection   303
Ischaemia, myocardial   45, 125

J wave   139
James by-pass   222

Katz-Wachtel phenomenon   292

Lead axis 106
Lead, Goldberger 312
Lead, Wilson 311
Leads, precordial 11
Left anterior hemiblock 119
Left axis deviation 116
Left bundle branch block 76
Left posterior hemiblock 120
Left ventricular hypertrophy 80
'Lone Auricular Fibrillation' 168
Low voltage, causes of 298
Lown-Ganong-Levine (L.G.L.)
     syndrome 242

Mahaim fibre 222
   pre-excitation 240
Mean electrical axis 111
Measurements 303
'Mirror-image dextrocardia 36, 115, 138,
   293
Mitral incompetence 290
Mitral stenosis 290
Mobitz Type I A-V block 210
Mobitz Type II A-V block 211
Myocardial infarction 298
   prognosis of 44
   vector principles 128
Myocardial injury 21
Myxoedema 68, 156

Necrosis, electrocardiographic
     manifestations of 19
Nodal rhythms *see* A-V nodal rhythms
Nomenclature of the electrode leads 6, 9
Non-pacemaking cell, action potential
     of 309
Non-paroxysmal A-V nodal
     tachycardia 175

Obstructive jaundice 156
Overdamping 299
Overdrive suppression 284
Overload concept 89
'Overshoot' 300

P. congenitale 137
P. pulmonale 137
P wave 101, 288
P wave axis 136
P wave retrograde 137
P waves absent 297
'P.A.T. with block' 164

P–R interval, measurement of 303
P–R interval, prolonged 207, 288
P–R interval, short 289
Pacemakers of the heart 148
   inherent discharge rate 148
Pacemaking cell, action potential
     of 310
Parasystole 201
Paroxysmal atrial tachycardia 163
Paroxysmal A-V nodal tachycardia 175
Paroxysmal ventricular
     tachycardia 186
Patent ductus arteriosus 292
Pericardial effusion 68
Pericarditis 65
Peri-infarction block 128
Phasic aberrant ventricular conduc-
     tion 258
Posterior infarction 30
Post-extrasystolic T wave change 65
Post-extrasystolic U wave inversion 65
Post-tachycardia syndrome 165
Potassium effect 95
'Premature atrial contraction' *see* Atrial
     extrasystoles
'Premature ventricular contraction' *see*
     Ventricular extrasystoles
Prinzmetal's angina 50
Pulmonary embolism 87
Pulmonary stenosis 291

Q wave, evaluation of 40
Q wave, pathological of myocardial
     infarction 19
Q wave, significance in Standard lead
     III 42
QRS complex 289
QRS-T angle 124
QRS-T relationship 54
Q–T interval 141, 303
Q–Tc 142
Quinidine effect 100

'R on T' phenomenon 188
Rate, determination of 147
Reciprocal rhythm 221
Reciprocating tachycardia 227, 230
   of W-P-W syndrome 237
Repolarization 304
Respiratory sinus arrhythmia 154
Retrograde atrial activation 105
Retrograde P wave 137
Rheumatic fever, acute 298
Rhythms, dual 151

Rhythms, fundamental aspects   150
Rhythms, reciprocal   221
Rhythms, secondary disorders   150
Right axis deviation   114
Right bundle branch block   36, 72
Right ventricular hypertrophy   83
'Rotation of the heart'   12
'Rule of Bigeminy'   183

S1, Q3, T3 pattern   85
S1, S2, S3 syndrome   84, 135
S-T segment   289
   coved of myocardial infarction   21, 22
Sick sinus syndrome   279
Sino-atrial (S-A) block   205
Sinus arrhythmia   154
Sinus bradycardia   155, 280
Sinus tachycardia   155, 280
Standard leads   107
Stokes-Adams attacks   213
Structural nodal disease   279
   aetiology   285
   evaluation   283
Summation complex *see* Fusion,
      ventricular
Supraventricular
      tachyarrhythmias   237
Supraventricular tachycardia   165, 228
Syncopal attack   213
Systolic overload   90

T wave   290
   change, extrasystolic   65
   effects, angina pectoris   53
T-VI taller thaj T-V6 syndrome   128
Tetralogy of Fallot   291

Transition zone   18, 298
Transmembrane action potential   309
Tricuspid atresia   291
Tricuspid stenosis   290

U wave   290
   in myocardial ischaemia   54
Underdamping   300
Unipolar leads   10, 109
   derivation of   310

Variant form of angina pectoris   50
Ventricular activation   5, 7
Ventricular activation time   303
Ventricular aneurysm   40
Ventricular asystole   213
Ventricular capture beat   252
Ventricular extrasystoles   179
   interpolated   183
Ventricular fibrillation   198
Ventricular flutter   195
   multiform   197
Ventricular fusion   191
   complexes   255
   mechanisms   257
Ventricular hypertrophy   80
Ventricular septal defect   292
Ventricular tachycardia   188
Vertical heart position   14

Wenckebach phenomenon   210
Wilson lead   311
Wolff-Parkinson-White (W-P-W)
      syndrome   36, 115, 117, 233
   fusion due to   257